Todd Family and Friends' Cookbook

Compiled and Edited
By Lewis and Linda Armstrong

Happy Cooking
Linda Armstrong
2017

Todd Family and Friends' Cookbook

DEDICATION

Dedicated to some of the best cooks in America at whose tables we have had the privilege of enjoying the foods they have prepared in years past. Especially to Irene (Woodell) Todd who was so loving and caring about her family. Her hand written recipes appear scattered within this cookbook.

CONTENTS

ACKNOWLEDGMENTS

The 5th Army and Fort Sam Houston 5th Wheels, Army wives for the recipes in a Cookbook we compiled and edited in 1994. The sisters at the church of Christ in Emporia, Kansas for recipes of the foods they prepared on Fridays at the Christian Student Center and for all the college students who enjoyed the food and fellowship. One student made a request for a cookbook with the recipes we had used on those Fridays so she could have them when she married. We did just that. She called us to let us know that one of the first meals she cooked, she used the cookbook. We compiled additional cookbooks with pictures and gave copies to six other students when they married. Then for the members of the Todd, Armstrong, friends, and neighbor families who contributed recipes we compiled a cookbook dedicated to Hubert and Irene Todd in 2007. Many recipes were from families' tables when we were children. It was in a loose leaf format and in three ring binders It included over 260 pictures of family members scattered throughout it and in the back a 'Family Matters' section with unique information about the Todd family and not included in this publication. We hope you enjoy this cookbook. Thanks for all the love and friendships you have shared with us through the years.

Also thank you to the artists at fiverr website for the artwork on the chapter pages.

Chapter 1

Appetizers and Snacks

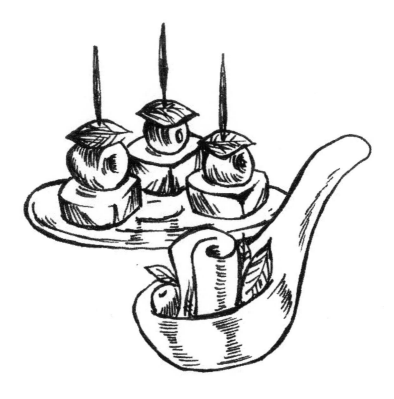

Index of Appetizer Recipes

Microwave Hot Oriental Chestnuts

½ c. soy sauce
½ tsp. ginger
Can water chestnuts cut into 1/3's
    or ½'s
Bacon slices, cut into thirds
    sugar

Combine all ingredients, except bacon and sugar, in a container and marinate in refrigerator for 2-4 hours. Wrap bacon around water chestnuts. Then roll in sugar. Place a few at a time on paper towel lined plate, cover with paper towel and microwave on HI until bacon is crispy. Cook 6 at a time for approximately 2½ minutes.

From the kitchen of Linda A.

The happiest people don't necessarily have the best of everything; they just make the most of everything that comes their way.

Microwave Fresh Vegetable Dippers

Fresh Vegetables:
    Mushrooms
    Broccoli
    Cauliflower
    Carrots
    Zucchini
Sauce:
1/3 c. margarine
¼ tsp. garlic powder
¼ - ½ tsp. seasoning salt
½ - 1 tbsp. lemon juice

Cut vegetables into equal sized parts. Mix sauce ingredients in 6 ounce bowl. Place on 12 inch glass plate. Arrange veggies around bowl. Cover bowl and tray tightly with two lengths of waxed paper, criss-crossed and edges tucked under the plate. For small amount, cook on HI for 4 – 4½ minutes or until tender crisp.

From the kitchen of Linda A.

Krazy Krunch

3 qt. air popped popcorn
Pkg. pecans
2 pkg. slivered almonds
2 sticks oleo
1½ c. sugar
½ c. white Karo syrup
1½ tbsp. vanilla
Stirring all the time, boil, until light caramel color between soft ball and firm ball stage. Add vanilla and stir popcorn. Then spread on wax paper that has been sprayed with Pam.
From the kitchen of Catherine G.

Microwave Pizza Cheese Snacks

1 lb. cheddar cheese, shredded
Large jar of pimentos
2 tbsp. minced onions
2 tbsp. oregano leaves
mayonnaise or salad dressing of choice
Stir ingredients together with enough mayonnaise to hold together. Spread on Triscuits or other crackers, place 6 on a plate and microwave for 15 seconds.
From the kitchen of Linda A.

"When God wants to speak and deal with us, he does not avail himself of an angel but of parents, of a friend, of a preacher, or of a neighbor." -- Martin Luther, 1483 – 1546, modified

Spinach Balls

2 boxes chopped frozen spinach, defrosted and water squeezed out
2 c. Pepperidge Farm herb stuffing mix
4 eggs, beaten
Stick butter, melted
½ c. grated parmesan cheese
½ - 1 tsp. garlic salt or garlic powder
½ tsp. black pepper
Mix all ingredients and form into 1 inch balls. Bake 20-25 minutes (until slightly brown) in 350 °F. oven. Makes 60 – 1 in. balls, serves 8. Freezes well (Make double batch and freeze one batch) Serve with spaghetti and sauce.
From the kitchen of Janet K.

Vegetable Pizza

2 pkg. crescent rolls
¼ c. red or green pepper,
    chopped, fine
¼ c broccoli, chopped, fine
¼ c. cauliflower, chopped, fine
¼ c. onions, chopped, fine
Pkg. Hidden Valley Ranch
    Dressing
2 – 8 oz. cream cheese
1 c. mayonnaise
Flatten crescent rolls on cookie
sheet (15½ inch x 10½ inch) Bake
at 400° F. for 8-10 minutes. Cool.
Mix cream cheese, mayonnaise,
and Ranch dressing. Spread
mixture on cool rolls and sprinkle
vegetables over top. Cut into small
squares and serve.
A Pampered Chef recipe,
submitted by Linda A.

A true friend is someone who
reaches for your hand and touches
your heart.

Black Bean Salsa

Ripe mango, peeled and diced
Red bell pepper, diced
Green bell pepper, diced
Red onion, diced
1 c. canned black beans, rinsed
1/3 c. pineapple juice
Juice of 2 limes
1 c. chopped cilantro
1 tbsp. ground cumin
1 tbsp. minced green chili pepper
    salt and pepper to taste
Combine first 10 ingredients in a
bowl. Season with salt and
pepper. Chill, covered for up to 5
days. Serve as a snack with
tortella chips.
From the kitchen of Janet K.

"I believe that maturity has more
to do with what types of
experiences you have had and
what you've learned from them
and less to do with how many
birthdays you've celebrated."

Barbecued Cocktail Wieners

1 c. catsup
1/3 c. Worcestershire sauce
1 tsp. chili powder
1/3 c. brown sugar
2 tbsp. vinegar
1 tbsp. liquid smoke
1½ c. water
½ tsp. salt
3 pkg. cocktail wieners

Combine all ingredients except wieners and heat to boiling point. Place the wieners in a baking dish, cover with liquid and cook in oven for 1 hour at 300 °F. Serve in a chafing dish or crock pot to keep them warm.
Makes 6 dozen.
From the kitchen of Mildred A.

Party Meatballs

1 lb. ground beef
2½ c. scalloped party crackers (Ritz) crushed
½ of a 4 oz. pkg. of creamy blue cheese
½ c. milk
½ tsp salt and pepper to taste

Small onion chopped fine (optional)
Garlic salt or use garlic powder (optional)
1 egg

Combine all ingredients except meat and let stand until softened. Add meat and mix well. Form into balls and broil 5-8 minutes. Makes about 18 large meatball or 35 small. If desired, the meatballs can be frozen. Let stand at room temperature for 35 minutes before cooking.
From the kitchen of Catherine G.

Cocktail Meatballs

2 lb. very lean ground beef
1 c. cornflakes, crushed
1/3 c. dried parsley flakes
2 eggs
2 tbsp. soy sauce
¼ tsp. pepper
½ tsp. garlic powder
2 tbsp. minced dried onion
1/3 c. catsup
One lb. can cranberry sauce
12 oz. bottle chili sauce
1 tbsp. firmly packed brown sugar
1 tbsp. lemon juice

Heat oven to 350° F. Combine

meat, cornflakes, parsley flakes, eggs, soy sauce, pepper, garlic powder, onion, and catsup. Blend well. Form into balls 1 inch. Diameter. Arrange in a large pan. In sauce pan, combine cranberry, chili sauce, brown sugar, and lemon juice. Cook on medium heat until cranberry sauce is melted. Pour over meat balls in pan. Bake uncovered 30 minutes. Serve in chafing dish with sauce. From the kitchen of Phyliss T.

Bacon Cups

10 count of biscuits
3 oz. jar real bacon bits
½ c. shredded parmesan cheese
8 oz softened cream cheese
Cut biscuit dough into thirds, put in mini-muffin tin and using finger, spread to form cup. Put mixture in the cups, bake at 350° F. for 12-14 minutes. Makes 30.
From the kitchen of Sally W.

"You are only young once, but you can be immature forever."

Peanut Butter Easter Eggs

2 lbs. powdered sugar
½ c. evaporated milk
2½ c. peanut butter
½ lb. margarine (2 sticks)
1 tsp. vanilla
Chocolate wafers
Mix all ingredients, except wafers, in large bowl. Knead until uniform consistency. Shape into small eggs. Put in refrigerator overnight or until firm. Then coat with melted chocolate wafers which you can find in the candy-making section at craft stores. Follow directions on wafer package about melting chocolate in microwave. When coating eggs with chocolate, suggest only removing 15 or 20 shaped eggs from the refrigerator at a time so the eggs don't get too soft before coating.
From the kitchen of June T.

Seven days without laughter makes one weak – Mort Walker

Coconut Easter Eggs

8 oz. package cream cheese
¼ lb. margarine
2 lbs. powdered sugar
7 oz. package flaked coconut
1 tsp. salt
1½ tsp. vanilla
chocolate wafers

Cream margarine and cheese together. Add sugar, salt, vanilla and coconut. Mix well. Put in refrigerator overnight before forming into eggs. [Before coating with chocolate, put shaped eggs into freezer to harden.] Coat with melted chocolate wafers which you can find in the candy-making section at craft stores. Follow directions on wafer package about melting chocolate in microwave. When coating eggs with chocolate, suggest only removing 15 or 20 shaped eggs from the freezer at a time so the eggs don't get too soft before coating.

From the kitchen of Patsy S.

"Age is important, only if you are cheese."

Boiled Custard

3 qt. milk
2¼ c. white sugar
6 eggs, well beaten
6 tbsp. cornstarch
1 tsp. vanilla

Fill the lower pan of a double boiler ⅓ full of water, and bring to a low boil. Pour milk into upper pot, and place over boiling water. Heat until small bubbles form around the edges of the milk. Stir in sugar, and continue stirring until it dissolves. In a small bowl, beat the eggs until light yellow. Remove about ½ cup hot milk, and gradually stir it into the eggs. Slowly mix the egg mixture into the milk in the pan. Mix in cornstarch; slowly stir into custard. Bring custard to a boil, and remove from heat. Stir in vanilla. Serve warm or chilled.

From the kitchen of Linda H.

Popcorn Balls

5 qt. popped corn
2 c. sugar
1½ c. water
½ tsp. salt
½ c. light corn syrup
1 tsp. vinegar
1 tsp. vanilla
Keep popcorn hot and crisp in low oven. (300° to 325° F.) Combine sugar, water, salt, corn syrup and vinegar. Cook to hard-ball stage (250° F.) Add vanilla. Pour slowly over popcorn. Mix well to coat every kernel. Use fat on hand, if necessary. Press into balls. Placing each one on a sheet of wax paper or a cookie sheet. Makes 15 -20 popcorn balls.
From the kitchen of Imodean D.

Let your virtues, if you have any, speak for their self. Refuse to talk about the vices of others.

Discourage gossip. It is a waste of valuable time and can be destructive and hurtful.

Tea Rings

2 pkg. yeast
¼ c. lukewarm water
1 c. milk
½ c. sugar
5 c. enriched flour
2 tsp. salt
¼ c. shortening
2 eggs
Soften yeast in lukewarm water. Scald milk. Add: sugar, salt, and shortening. Cool to lukewarm. Add flour to make a thicker batter, mix well. Add enough flour to make a soft dough. Turn out on lightly floured board and knead until smooth and satiny. Place in greased bowl, cover, let rise in a warm place until doubled (about 1½ hours) when light, punch down and then let rest 10 minutes. Shape into rings. Let rise until doubled (about 1 hour) Bake in oven at 350° F. for 30 minutes.
From the kitchen of Imodean D.

Since it's the early worm that gets eaten by the bird, sleep late.

Cheese Ball

2 – 8 oz. pkg. cream cheese (softened)
6 – 7 sm. Green onions
2 fresh Serrano peppers
2 – 2.5 oz. pkg. sliced cooked beef (Buddig Brand)
2 med. Size fresh jalapeno pepper
¾ tsp. garlic salt

Chop onions and peppers in chopper of food processor until finely chopped. Chop beef in chopper of food processor until finely chopped. Blend cream cheese, onion and pepper mixture and about ¾ of the chopped beef until well blended. Add garlic salt to taste (about ¾ teaspoon.) and mix well. With hands, form two small or one large ball. Use the remaining ¼ chopped beef to cover the outside of the cheese ball. Refrigerate overnight in order to set firmly. Enjoy with Town House Cracker.

From the kitchen of Debbie W.

Imodean's Hush Puppies

1 c. corn meal
2 tsp. baking powder
1 c. flour
½ tsp. salt
1 egg
milk-just enough to mix

Mix together the dry ingredients, then add the egg and the milk as needed. With a stiff consistency, roll into 1 inch balls, place on a cookie sheet and bake at 400° F for 15 minutes.

From the kitchen of Imodean D.

"In everyone's life, at some time, our inner fire goes out. It is then burst into flame by an encounter with another human being. We should all be thankful for those people who rekindle the inner spirit." – Albert Schweitzer

Chapter 2
Beverages

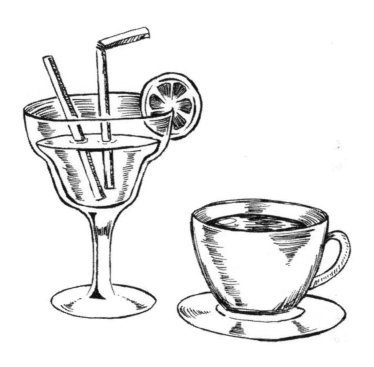

Index of Beverage Recipes

Special Occasion Punch

Small pkg. orange jello
Small pkg. apricot jello
4 c. boiling water
1½ c. sugar
46 oz. can pineapple juice, cold
2 c. cold water
Liter ginger ale, cold
½ gallon lime sherbet
Stir the jello in the boiling water till dissolved. Add and stir in the sugar and cold water. Refrigerate till ready to serve. Just before serving, put in punch bowl and add pineapple juice, sherbet, and ginger ale.
Unknown kitchen.

Lucille's Punch

2 pkg. Koolaid, any flavor you wish
1¼ c. sugar, Splenda or Stevia
46 oz. can pineapple juice.
8 oz. can orange juice, thawed
2 liter bottle of ginger ale
Mix everything but ginger ale and freeze. Take out of freezer 1 hour before serving. Put in a punch bowl. Mash with potato masher. Should be kind of slushy. Add cold ginger ale and serve. Makes 121 ounces (15 cups) enough for a punch bowl.
From the kitchen of Lucille D.

"Let your daily exercise be your walk with God."

Wedding Punch

6 oz. can frozen orange juice concentrate
6 oz. can frozen lemonade concentrate
12 oz. can apricot nectar
2 can (2½ c.) pineapple juice
Add water to the frozen concentrates as directed on cans. Combine with apricot nectar and pineapple juice. Chill. Serve in punch bowl.
Float block of ice in punch. Garnish with orange slices. Serves 24. Makes 3 quart. Double or triple recipe if needed.
From unknown kitchen.

Punch

Can frozen lemonade
4 cans water
2 large boxes of strawberry jello
3 c. sugar or less, (just to taste)
2 c. hot water.
46 oz. can orange juice
42 oz. can pineapple juice
Dissolve the jello with the hot water then mix all the ingredients and refrigerate for 2-4 hours. At last minute, add a two liter bottle of ginger ale and serve.
From unknown kitchen.

Wedding Punch for Melba's Wedding

Large can pineapple juice
2 lg. can High-C Orange Drink
About 4 lb. sugar or to taste
1 doz. lemons squeezed into juice
4 pkg. strawberry jello dissolved in 2 c. boiling water.
Add enough water to make 4 full gallons. Chill. Just before serving, 1 liter bottle of cold ginger ale.
From the kitchen of Irene T.

Green Punch

6 pkg. Lemon lime powder cool-aid
3 c. sugar and
3 qts. water
Large can of pineapple juice (32 oz.)
Liter of ginger ale
Stir mixture well before serving.
From the kitchen of Melba R.

Spiced Tea

½ c. sugar
2 c. water
1 tsp. Whole cloves
Stick cinnamon
Simmer above ingredients on stove for 10 minutes. Remove cloves and cinnamon.
Add:
Large can of frozen orange juice
Small can of frozen lemonade
4 c. of very strong tea. (Use 8 small tea bags when brewing.)
From the kitchen of Linda A.

"If you're headed in the wrong direction, God allows U-turns."

Microwave Spiced Cider

1/3 c. brown sugar
1/3 c. water
2 tbsp. whole cloves
2 sticks cinnamon
1 tbsp. whole allspice
¼ tsp. salt
2 qt. cider
1 c. orange juice
Put sugar, water and seasoning in a 4 cup measure. Microwave on HI 4 - 6 minutes to form a light syrup. Combine with cider and orange juice in 3 quart casserole dish. Microwave on HI 7 to 9 minutes until heated. Strain before serving.

From the kitchen of Linda A.

Hot Chocolate Mix

1 lb. Quik Chocolate mix
8 qt. box powdered milk
Stir together and store in a large jar or canister. Fill the mug you are using about ½ full of the mix. Fill with boiling or very hot water and stir well and serve. Add marshmallows if desired. Makes a good gift in a jar. Makes about 50 servings.
From the kitchen of Linda A.

WARNING: Exposure to the Son may prevent burning.

A Great Recipe

Fold two hands together, and express a dash of sorrow.

Marinate it overnight, and work on it tomorrow.

Chop one grudge in tiny pieces, add several cups of love.

Dredge with a large sized smile, mix with the ingredients above.

Dissolve the hate within you, by doing a good deed.

Cut in and help your friend, if he/she should be in need.

Stir in laughter, love and kindness, from the heart it has to come.

Toss with genuine forgiveness, and give your friends some.

The amount of people served, will depend on you.

It can serve the whole wide world. If you really want it to! author unknown

Chapter 3
Breads and Rolls

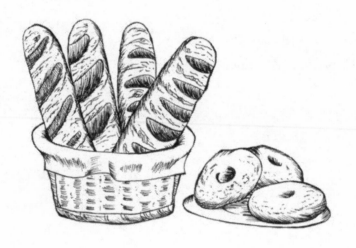

Index For Bread and Roll Recipes

Biscuits

2 c. flour
4 tsp. baking powder
½ tsp. salt
½ tsp. cream of tartar
2 tsp. sugar
½ c. shortening
2/3 c. milk

Combine together dry ingredients. Cut shortening into dry ingredients and combine with the milk. Roll and cut out biscuits or spoon out and drop biscuits on cookie sheet. Bake at 450° F. to desired doneness. Makes 12 -14 biscuits.
From the kitchen of Bobbye P.

All American Waffles

2 eggs, separated
1¾ c. milk
¼ c. vegetable oil
1¾ c. flour
2 tbsp. sugar
4 tsp. baking powder
1 tsp. salt

Beat egg yolks, stir in milk and oil. Add flour, sugar, baking powder and salt. Stir just until large lumps disappear. Beat egg white until stiff and gently fold into batter for light fluffy waffles. Bake and serve.
From the kitchen of Aukse H.

Biscuit Mix

20 c. flour
¾ c. + 4 tsp. baking powder
3 tbsp. plus 1 tsp. salt
3⅓ c. shortening

Mix well above ingredients. When preparing batch, add milk as needed. Use 5 cups to make biscuits for a meal.
From the kitchen of Mildred A.

Remember the five simple rules to be happy:

1. Free your heart from hatred.
2. Free your mind from worries.
3. Live simply.
4. Give more.
5. Expect less.

Waffles

1¾ c. flour
1 tbsp. baking powder
1 tsp. salt
2 eggs
1¼ c. milk
6 tbsp. cooking oil (¼ c. plus 2
    tbsp.)

Measure and sift the flour, baking powder and sugar. Beat the eggs. Mix together the eggs, milk and cooking oil. Mix in the dry ingredients. Pour into waffle maker. Makes up to eight waffles.
From the kitchen of Melba R.

Garlic Bread

½ c. soft butter (¼ lb.)
¼ c. parmesan cheese (grated)
2 tsp. fresh parsley
1 tsp. Giroy Farms crushed garlic or
    2 cloves chopped fine
1 tsp. oregano

Combine all ingredients in a bowl and mix well. Slice a loaf of French or Italian bread in 1 inch slices. Spread garlic mixture between slices. Place in foil and seal. Bake on baking sheet 12 - 15 minutes in a preheated 350° F. oven OR slice a loaf of French or Italian bread horizontally. Spread garlic mixture on each half. Place under a broiler. Watch closely for preferred toasted appearance.
From the kitchen of Linda A.

Yeast Rolls

1 c. boiling water
1 c. Crisco
¾ c. sugar
1-2 tsp. salt
2 pkg. dry yeast
1 c. cold water
5-6 c. flour
2 eggs (beaten)

Pour boiling water over Crisco, sugar and salt. Blend and cool. Add beaten eggs. Soak yeast in cold water and add to the mixture. Add flour by stirring and kneading, then oil top, cover and refrigerate immediately. About 1½ to 2 hours before using, remove from the refrigerator. Make out rolls and dip in butter. Let rise. Bake at 375-400° F. until the desired doneness. (This dough will last in the refrigerator for several days)
From the kitchen of Bobbye P.

Challah Bread

Dissolve:
1½ pkg. of rapid rise yeast
1½ c. warm water
Combine:
2 eggs, beaten
½ c. oil
¾ c. sugar
¾ tsp salt
Add to yeast and water mixture.
Start adding about 6 cups flour.
Next knead until it feels right and is
smooth. Put in large bowl. Oil top
and cover. Let rise until double in
size. Punch down, form loaves and
put in 2 loaf pans, cover and let rise.
Brush top with a beaten egg to glaze
it and sprinkle with poppy or
sesame seeds. Bake 40 minutes at
350 ° F.
From the kitchen of Michou A.

Prayer is not a 'spare wheel' that you
pull out when in trouble; it is a
'steering wheel' that directs us in the
right path throughout life.

Mother's Cornbread Recipe

Cornbread

Sift together
1½ C meal
½ C flour
½ t salt
½ t baking powder

add
1 egg
1½ C milk

mix & pour into a heated pan
& bake till brown.

From the kitchen of Irene T.

Corn Bread (Sweet)

1 c. flour
3 tsp. baking powder
½ tsp. salt
½ c. sugar
½ c. cornmeal
1 c. milk
1 egg
1 tbsp. shortening, melted
Mix dry ingredients then stir in milk,
egg, and the shortening. Bake at
400° F. for 20 minutes.
From the kitchen of Kim T.

Spoon Bread

2 c. cornmeal
1½ c. sweet potatoes, mashed
2 c. boiling water
1 tsp. salt
3 tbsp. butter, melted
3 eggs

Sift the cornmeal three times and dissolve with potatoes in the boiling water. Mix until smooth and free from any lumps. Add melted butter and salt. Thin with milk. Separate the eggs. Beat yolks to the mixture, then beat and add the whites. Pour into baking dish and bake in 350° F. oven for 30 minutes or until done.
From the kitchen of Ethel A.

Buttermilk Cornbread

2 c. cornmeal
2 tsp. baking powder
1 tsp. salt and 1 tsp. sugar
½ tsp. baking soda
3 tbsp. shortening
1½ c. buttermilk
2 eggs

Mix cornmeal, baking powder, salt, baking soda, and sugar in a bowl. Melt shortening. Add buttermilk, eggs and shortening to the cornmeal mixture and beat well. Fill greased pan half full and bake at 425° F. (hot oven) for 15-20 minutes until browned on top. Cut into squares and serve at once.
From the kitchen of Ethel A.

Bran Refrigerator Muffins

2 c. 100% Bran
Pour 2 c. boiling water over the Bran and let cool while preparing the following:
1 c. shortening creamed
3 c. sugar or (½ c. canola oil creamed ½ c. applesauce with 3 c. Splenda)
Add 4 beaten eggs &
1 qt. buttermilk.
Sift together:
5 c. flour (may use part whole wheat)
5 tsp. soda and 1 tsp. salt

Add the dry ingredients with the bran mixture to the creamed ingredients. Then add 4 cups All-bran. Mix only till moistened. Store in quart jars in your refrigerator. Bake as wanted for 12 minutes at 400° F. Makes about 4 quarts and keeps up to 4 weeks. (You may wish to cook and freeze some or all of the muffins instead.)
From the kitchen of Linda A.

19

Sweet Banana Bread

½ c. butter

1½ c. granulated sugar

2 eggs, beaten

½ c. buttermilk

2 c. flour

1½ tsp. baking soda

¼ tsp. baking powder

¾ c. pecans, chopped

1 c. ripe banana pulp (2 large bananas)

1 tsp. vanilla

Cream together the butter and sugar. Add beaten eggs and buttermilk. Sift together the flour, baking soda and baking powder and add this to the sifted ingredients. Stir in the pecans, banana pulp and vanilla. Turn into a greased 9 inch x 3 inch x 2 inch loaf pan and bake at 350° F. for about an hour. Or use two 8 inch or 9 inch round layer cake pans and make a layer cake instead of a loaf.

From the kitchen of Mildred A.

Banana - Bran Muffins

2 tbsp. tofu

Egg replacement of 1 egg

3 large ripe bananas (1½ c.)

3 tbsp. sunflower oil

1/3 c. honey or maple syrup

Dash of salt (optional)

1 c. whole wheat pastry flour

1 tbsp. soy flour

Scant ¾ c. oat bran

2 tsp. baking powder

½ tsp. baking soda

1 tsp. ground cinnamon

½ tsp. ground nutmeg

1. Preheat oven to 375° F. With a hand blender or in a food processor, cream tofu, egg replacement, bananas, oil and sweetener.

2. In a separate bowl, combine salt, flour, oat bran, baking powder, baking soda, cinnamon and nutmeg. Make a well in the center and add banana mixture, folding in with a spatula until dry ingredients are thoroughly moistened.

3. Oil 10 - 12 muffin cups, depending on the desired size. Spoon batter into cups and bake for 20-25 minutes or until muffin are lightly browned and a toothpick inserted in the center comes out clean. Cool briefly and turn out to finish cooling on a wire rack.

From the kitchen of Michou A.

Cranberry Bread

2 c. sifted flour
1½ tsp. baking soda
½ tsp. salt
1 c. sugar
1 c. chopped nuts
1 orange rind, grated
1 egg, beaten
1 c. cranberries, raw, quartered

Sift ingredients together, then mix with nuts, orange rind and cranberries. In a measuring cup, put 2 tablespoon of Crisco and juice of one orange. Fill cup with boiling water. Stir into mixture adding eggs last. Bake 1 hour at 325° F. in loaf pan.

From the kitchen of Ethel A.

Honey of a Date Bread

1 tbsp. orange rind, grated
½ c. orange juice
½ c. honey
2 c. cornmeal, self rising
1 c. dates, pitted, chopped
1 c. nuts, finely chopped
3 eggs, beaten
1 to 1¼ c. milk
¼ c. oil
2 tbsp. honey

In a small sauce pan combine orange rind, orange juice and the ½ cup honey. Simmer, stirring occasionally, about 15 minutes. In a medium bowl, stir together cornmeal, dates and nuts. Blend eggs, milk, oil and honey add all at once in cornmeal mixture, stirring until smooth. If necessary, add more milk to make a medium thick batter. Pour into greased 9 inch round baking pan. Pour orange and honey mixture over the top. Gently run knife through the batter to marble honey mixture through. Bake at 425° F. for 25 to 30 minutes or until golden brown. Cut in wedges and serve with ice cream. Serves 6-8.

From the kitchen of Ethel A.

Be Kind

Be kind to others, for I love them just as much as I love you. They may not dress like you, or talk like you, or live the same way you do, but I still love you all. Please try to get along, for My sake. I created each of you different in some way. It would be too boring if you were all identical. Please, know I love each of your differences.

Author unknown

Date Nut Bread

1 c. dates, cut in pieces
1 c. boiling water
1 c. sugar
1 egg beaten
1 tbsp. butter or margarine
1 7/8 c. flour
2/3 tsp. salt
2/3 tsp. baking soda
2/3 tsp. cream of tartar
1 tsp. vanilla
1/3 c. nuts, chopped
Mix dates, boiling water, sugar, and butter. When cool, add remaining ingredients and mix well. Bake in a loaf pan for 1 hour at 350° F.
From the kitchen of Mildred A.

Whiz Nut Bread

½ c. sugar
1 egg
1¼ c. milk
3 c. Bisquick
1½ c. chopped nuts
Mix in a bowl sugar, egg, milk, and the Bisquick. Beat hard for 30 seconds. After mixing, stir in nuts. Grease thoroughly a 9 inch loaf pan. Pour into loaf pan. Bake at 350° F. for 45 - 50 minutes.
From the kitchen of Mildred A.

No God, No Peace; Know God, Know Peace

Pumpkin Bread

1 c. shortening
3 eggs
#303 can pumpkin
2½ c. sugar
½ tsp. baking powder
3½ c. flour
1 tsp. baking soda
1 tsp. cinnamon
1 tsp. nutmeg
1 tsp. allspice
1 tsp. cloves
½ c. chopped nuts
Mix shortening, eggs and pumpkin. In a separate bowl, combine dry ingredients. Add to pumpkin mixture and blend well. Add nuts and stir. Pour into two greased, floured loaf pans and bake at 325°F for one hour. Let cool before removing from pans.
From the kitchen of Mildred A.

Old friends are like Gold! New friends are Diamonds! If you get a Diamond, don't forget the Gold! Because to hold a Diamond, you always need a base of Gold.

Pumpkin Bread

3½ c. flour
2 tsp. baking soda
½ tsp. salt
1 tsp. cinnamon
3 c. sugar
½ c. nuts
4 eggs
1 c. oil
½ c. water
2 c. pumpkin

Dredge nuts in flour. Combine dry ingredients. Beat eggs well, add oil and pumpkin. Mix dry ingredients with the liquid. Bake at 350°F. for 1¼ hours.

From the kitchen of Ethel A.

Elderberry Bread

3¾ c. rye flour
1 ⅓ c. barley flour, or 1 ⅓ c. any
    whole-grain flour
5 tbsp. freshly ground flaxseeds
1 tsp. baking soda
½ tsp. salt
3¼ c. apple juice or other
    unsweetened fruit juice
2 tbsp. corn oil
1 tsp. coconut extract (optional)
1 tsp. amaretto extract (optional)
2 c. elderberries
1 c. granola
1 c. shelled raw sunflower seeds
1 c. unsweetened shredded coconut
2 tbsp. lecithin granules
1 tsp. ground cinnamon

Preheat the oven to 350°F. Mix the flour, ground flaxseeds, baking soda, and salt in a large bowl. In a medium-size bowl, mix together the apple juice, liquid stevia, if you are using it, lemon juice, corn oil, and extracts. Mix the wet ingredients into the dry ingredients, being careful not to over mix. Stir in the elderberries, granola, sunflower seeds, coconut, and lecithin. Press the dough into 2 oiled 8½ inch x 4 ½ inch x 2½ inch bread pans. Sprinkle the cinnamon on top. Set a pan of hot water on the bottom of the oven to keep the crust soft. Bake the loaves until a toothpick inserted in the center emerges clean, about 1 hour. Remove the loaves from the oven and let them cool on a wire rack before slicing.

Adapted from *The Wild Vegetarian Cookbook,* by 'Wildman' Steve Brill (Harvard Common Press, 2002).

Pineapple Bread

¼ lb. butter
1 c. sugar
4 eggs
20 oz. can crushed pineapple
5 to 7 slices of white bread, cubed
Mix butter, sugar and eggs together. Add pineapple and cubed bread. Pour into 1½ quart casserole dish and bake at 350° F. for 30 – 35 minutes.

Fort Larimore Army Bread Recipe

(Bulk Recipe)

9 c. water
13 c. flour, un-sifted
2 tbsp. powdered yeast
2 tbsp. salt
Into a bowl, pour 4 cups of lukewarm water. Dissolve the yeast, then mix in 4 cups of flour. Let sponge sit covered with a towel in a warm place, for 1 hour. Then add 5 more cups lukewarm water, salt -7 cup to 9 cup cut flour till doughy consistency is reached. Mix well, kneading in bowl. Set aside in warm place for 1 hour, covered. Return and knead dough on a flat lightly floured surface. Return to bowl, coat surface with lard and set aside for 1 hour. Then knead dough lightly, cut into 20 ounce loaves. Place into greased pans, coating loaves again lightly with lard. Cover and let rise. When sufficiently risen, place pans in oven preheated to 400° F. for 30-45 minutes or until golden brown. Remove, coat freshly baked bread with lard. It makes approximately, 8 – 18 ounce loaves.

This Recipe is adapted from 'Practical Instructions in Breadmaking,' GPO Washington, DC. 1878.
From the kitchen of Susan M.

Basic Sweet Dough

2 pkg. yeast
¼ c. warm water
1 c. milk
½ c. sugar
½ tsp. salt
5 c. enriched flour
¼ c. shortening
2 eggs
Dissolve yeast in lukewarm water. Scald milk and add sugar, salt, shortening. Cool to lukewarm. Add flour to make a thick batter.

Add yeast and eggs. Beat well. Add more flour to have a good consistency.

From the kitchen of Ethel A.

Sweet Dough

(Bulk Recipe)

8 oz. shortening
8 oz. sugar
½ oz. salt
2 oz. powdered milk
¼ oz. malt
3 eggs
1 lb. water
2 oz. yeast
2 lb. + 4 oz. bread flour

From the Skirvin Tower Hotel, Oklahoma City, OK, 1960.

Sweet Dough

1½ c. lukewarm milk
½ c. sugar
2 tsp. salt
2 pkg. dry yeast
½ c. warm water
2 eggs
½ c. oil
Chives
7 to 7½ c. flour

Mix sugar and salt into the warm milk. Dissolve the dry yeast in warm water. Add the milk. Add eggs, oil and chives and mix good. Now start adding flour. Add enough to make a dough easy to handle - where it is no longer sticky. Turn out on floured board. Knead. Now put under pan to rest 10 minutes. Work down. Now put in greased pan or bowl to rise. After 2nd rising, make into rolls. Bake at 350 - 375° F. Can use this for pull apart bread, cinnamon rolls - all kinds of sweet breads and rolls.

From the kitchen of Catherine G.

Broccoli Cornbread

Combine and microwave until tender
10 oz. broccoli, cut up and 1 stick butter or margarine
Large onion, chopped
Mix together
16 oz. container cottage cheese
2 Jiffy onion broth mix
4 eggs
Stir in broccoli mixture
Bake 40-45 minutes at 325° F. in a 9 inch x 13 inch grease pan.

From the kitchen of Selma L.

Sunday Dinner Rolls

Pkg. active dry yeast
1 c. warm water
½ c. cooking oil
4 c. all- purpose flour
1 tsp. salt
½ c. sugar
2 eggs, lightly beaten
In a large bowl, dissolve yeast in warm water. Add oil, flour, salt, sugar, and eggs, mixing thoroughly. Cover and let stand 8 hr. or overnight. Roll ½ inch thick, cut into rolls. Place on greased cookie sheet. Let rise 4 to 6 hours. Preheat oven to 400° F. Bake 10-12 minutes. Suggest making the dough on Saturday and make the rolls Sunday morning before going to worship.
From the kitchen of Evelyn B.

Ezekiel 4:9 Bread

2½ c. wheat berries
1½ c. spelt flour
½ c. barley
½ c. millet
¼ c. dry green lentils
2 tbsp. dry great Northern beans
2 tbsp. dry kidney beans
2 tbsp. dried pinto beans
4 c. warm water (110° F)
1 c. honey
½ c. olive oil
2 - .25 oz. pkg. active dry yeast
1 tsp. salt
Measure the water, honey, olive oil, and yeast into a large bowl. Let sit for 3 to 5 minutes. Stir all of the grains and beans together until well mixed. Grind in a flour mill. Add fresh milled flour and salt to the yeast mixture; stir until well mixed, about 10 minutes. The dough will be like that of a batter bread. Pour dough into two greased 9 inch x 5 inch loaf pans. Let rise in a warm place for about 1 hour, or until dough has reached the top of the pan.   Bake at 350° F for 45 to 50 minutes, or until loaves are golden brown. "Take thou also unto thee wheat, and barley, and beans, and lentils, and millet, and spelt, and put them in one vessel, and make thee bread thereof;…" Ezekiel 4:9a
From the kitchen of Susan M.

Hard Rolls & Sticks

(Bulk Recipe)

2 qt. water
½ lb. yeast
½ pt. egg whites
2 oz. sugar
2 oz. salt
2 oz shortening
¼ oz yeast food
5 lb. flour
2½ lb. upheaval
Scale - 3 lb. for hard rolls
     - 2 lb. + 4 oz for sticks
Cook for 23 minutes for 400° - 410°F.
From the Skirvin Tower Hotel, Oklahoma City, OK, 1960.

Fruit Muffins

(Bulk Recipe)

1 qt. fruit, chopped fine
1 lb. sugar
1 lb. Tastex shortening, colored
    yellow with butter flavor
1 oz. salt
8 eggs
1½ qt. milk
3 lb. bread flour
1 lb. cake flour
4 oz. baking powder
14 dozen fruit
From the Skirvin Tower Hotel, Oklahoma City, OK, 1960.

Orange Muffins

(Bulk Recipe)

2½ c. soft wheat
2½ c. hard wheat
5 oz. baking powder
1 lb. + 5 oz shortening
1 oz. salt
½ gal. milk.
2 eggs
1½ oz. yeast
Dissolve in liquid
2 large oranges, grated
Squeeze juice, rest beater, add eggs and yeast
From the Skirvin Tower Hotel, Oklahoma City, OK, 1960.

Delicious Easy Rolls

1 box yellow cake mix
5 c. flour
2 pkg. yeast
2½ c. warm water
1¼ tsp. salt
Dissolve yeast in 1 c. warm water and let stand until dissolved. Pour flour in large bowl, not plastic. Add cake mix and stir together. Then add remaining warm water, salt and yeast mixture. Stir well, then knead and let rise in bulk. Knead down and make into rolls or cinnamon

rolls. Place on four 9 inch pans. Bake 20 minutes or until brown at 350° F.

From the kitchen of Mildred A.

Ice Box Rolls

1 qt. sweet milk
1 c. shortening
¾ c. sugar
1 cake yeast
1 tsp. soda
2 tsp. salt
2 qt. flour
2 tsp. baking powder

Scald milk (do not boil) with the shortening and sugar. Let cool to luke warm, then crumble in the yeast, stirring to dissolve. Add 1 quart. flour and beat hard with a rotary beater until smooth as cake dough. Let rise in warm place until double in bulk. Cut down with a spoon and add the remaining ingredients. More flour may be added if needed. Pour out onto a well floured board and knead at least 10 minutes. Do not use anymore flour that necessary. Place in a well greased crock or pan; grease top of dough. Cover with wax paper and set in refrigerator until needed. Cut off the amount of dough wanted; roll out and cut into

any kind of rolls you want. Let rise until very light. Bake in a quick oven. Dough will keep in the refrigerator for several days.

From the kitchen of Imodean D.

No-Knead Refrigerator Rolls

2 cubes fresh yeast
2 c. very warm water (105° to 115° F.)
½ c. sugar
1½ tsp. salt
7 c. all-purpose flour
1 egg, beaten
¼ c. solid Crisco shortening

In a large bowl, place yeast in the water, and let stand 5 min. to dissolve. Add the egg, shortening, sugar, salt. Then mix in the flour, and beat until smooth, Cover with a damp cloth and let rise in refrigerator. Punch down and replace damp cloth. About 2 hr. before serving, grease a baking sheet. Cut off as much dough as you need and shape into small rolls. Place the rolls on the baking sheet, cover with waxed paper and a kitchen towel and let rise until double in size - about 1½ hours. Heat oven to 400° F. and bake for

12- 15 minutes. Makes 36 to 40.
From the *Feingold Cookbook for Rolls*
From the kitchen of Imodean D.

Rolls I

½ c. sugar
¼ c. melted oleo
2 eggs
¼ tsp. salt
2 c. warm water
3 pkg. dry yeast
6 c. flour
Dissolve yeast in the warm water.
In another bowl, beat sugar and
butter, and add eggs and salt. Beat
until smooth. Add yeast mixture to
this. Add 3 cup flour a little at a
time. Let set for 5 minutes. Add
the rest of the flour, a little at a time.
Make into rolls. Bake at 400° F.
about 20 minutes.
From the kitchen of Mildred A.

Life is not measured by the number
of breaths we take; but by the
moments that take our breath away!

Rolls II

4 c. sweet milk
1 c. shortening
¾ c. sugar
1 cake yeast
1 tsp. baking soda
2 tsp salt
2 tsp. baking powder
8 c. flour
Scald milk (Do not boil) with the
shortening and sugar. Let cool to
lukewarm, then crumble in the
yeast, stirring to dissolve. Add 1
quart of the flour and beat hard
with a rotary beater until smooth as
cake dough. Let rise in warm place
until double in bulk. Cut down with
a spoon and add remaining
ingredients. More flour may be
added if needed. Pour out onto a
well floured board and knead for at
least 10 minutes.   Do not use any
more flour than necessary. Place in
a well greased crock or pan. Grease
top of dough, cover with a wax
paper; and set in refrigerator. Cut
off the amount of dough wanted.
Bake at 400° F. for 20 minutes.
From the kitchen of Mildred A.

Yeast Starter

3 potatoes (¾ lb.)
1¼ c. boiling water
4 tbsp. sugar
1½ tsp. salt
1½ c. cold water
1 cake compress yeast
Use good, sound, clean potatoes. Peel, wash, and cut them into small pieces and cook until tender in the boiling water.   Mash the potatoes in the water in which they were cooked.   Add sugar, salt and enough cold water to make 3¼ cups of liquid and allow this mixture to become lukewarm (about 82°). Dissolve the cake compressed yeast in 1 cup lukewarm water and add to the lukewarm mixture. Allow this mixture to stand overnight. In the morning it should be light and frothy and is ready to use. Stir it well. Pour off one cup to save as starter for the next baking and store it in a clean, scalded jar, loose cover, in a cool place. Keep from freezing. From the kitchen of Bobbye P.

Poor Boy

(Bulk Recipe)

7 lb. flour
7 lb. upheaval
4 oz. salt
4 oz. dry Niamalt
4 oz. shortening
2 oz. sugar
1 oz. yeast food
3½ qt. water
1 pt. egg whites
12 oz. Fleishman's yeast
From the Skirvin Tower Hotel, Oklahoma City, Oklahoma, 1960.

There are five things that you cannot recover in life!!

(1) The Stone...after it's thrown,
(2) The Word...after it's said,
(3) The Occasion...after it's missed.
(4) The Time...after it's gone, and
(5) A Person...after they die.

Talk To Me

I want you to forget a lot of things.
Forget what was making you crazy.
Forget the worry and the fretting
because you know I'm in control.
But there's one thing I pray you
never forget.   Please, don't forget
to talk to Me - OFTEN! I love
YOU! I want to hear your voice.   I
want you to include Me in on the
things going on in your life. I want
to hear you talk about your friends
and family.   Prayer is simply you
having a conversation with Me.   I
want to be your dearest friend.
Author unknown

Chapter 4

Dips, Dressings, Sauces, Gravies, Toppings and Spreads

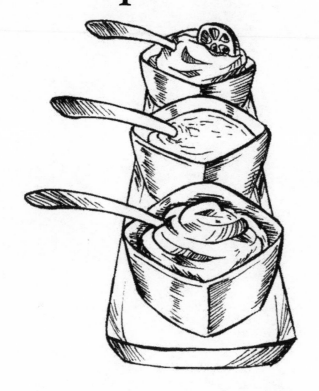

Index of Dip etc. Recipes

California Guccamole Dip

2 c. sour cream
1 envelope onion soup mix
½ c. chopped green pepper
1 medium tomato, chopped
1 avocado, mashed
1 tsp. lemon juice
¼ tsp. garlic powder
Combine all ingredients. Chill. Serve with slices strips of vegetables such as carrots, celery, cucumber, radishes, green peppers, etc.
From the kitchen of Paula H.

Catherine's Cheesy Artichoke Dip

Can (14 oz.) artichoke hearts, drained and chopped *I use 2 cans!
1 c. mayonnaise
1 c. (4 oz.) shredded mozzarella cheese
1 c. grated Parmesan cheese, divided
1 tbsp. chopped onion
1 tbsp. minced fresh parsley
¼ tsp. garlic salt
2 -3 fresh artichokes, optional assorted crackers
Combine artichoke hearts, mayo,

mozzarella, ½ cup Parmesan, onion, parsley and garlic salt. Spoon into ungreased one quart baking dish. Top with remaining Parmesan cheese. Bake uncovered at 350° F. for 20 minutes. If desired, use fresh artichokes as serving bowls. Remove the center leaves, leaving a hollow shell; spoon dip into shell. Serve warm with crackers. Makes 16 servings.
From the kitchen of Catherine G.

New Year Eve Party Dip

Cream Together:
2 large pkg. Neuchâtel Cream Cheese, softened
20 oz. can crushed pineapple in own juice, drained (use ½ of juice)
Stir In:
½ c. onion, chopped
1 c. pecans, chopped
½ c. celery, chopped
1 c. shredded cheese
Use with crackers, veggies, etc.
From the kitchen of Elaine S.
Make promises sparingly and keep them faithfully, no matter what the cost.

Cheese Dip

2 lbs. American Cheese (Blue Box)
2 to 3 stocks of celery, finely
  chopped
2 cans chopped green chiles
2 cans Rotel
Onion to taste, finely chopped
Combine all ingredients in sauce
pan or slow cooker. Cook until easy
to spread.
From the kitchen of Debbie W.

Hot Bean Dip

2 tbsp. tomato juice or V-8 juice
1 tsp. garlic salt or ½ tsp. garlic
  powder
2 tbsp. vinegar
2 tsp. Worcestershire sauce
1 tsp. chili powder
No. 2½ can pork & beans (3½ c.)
Dash cayenne
Put these ingredients in a blender
and blend at high speed till smooth
or mash with a fork.
May have to blend in two batches.
Prepare:
½ c. cubed, processed American
  cheese
4 slices bacon; fried crisp, crumbled
Add the cheese and bacon to
blended mixture and heat in a
baking dish or chafing dish till

cheese melts. Stir. Serve hot with
celery sticks, broccoli, and/or
carrots.
From the kitchen of Linda A.

Sweet and Sour Dressing

¼ c. oil
2 tbsp. sugar
2 tbsp. vinegar
1 tbsp. parsley
½ tsp. salt
dash of pepper
dash of red pepper
Mix ingredients and serve with
salad.
From the kitchen of Catherine G.

Cattleman's Dressing

1 qt. Kraft Mayonnaise (or Hellman's)
Lg. can Milnot
2 tsp. garlic powder
2 tbsp. fresh lemon juice
1 c. grated American Cheese
2 tbsp. Worchester Sauce
1 tsp. sugar
Mix all in a blender and store in the refrigerator.
From the kitchen of Gert S.

Seven Layer Chalupa Dip

16 oz. can refried beans (reg. or jalapeño)
9 oz. can bean dip (reg. or jalapeño)
8 oz. cartoon sour cream (light or fat free can be used as well.
2 tbsp. mayonnaise (reg., lite, or fat-free)
3 tbsp. Picante sauce
3 lg. avocados, mashed
salt and pepper to taste
1 tsp. lemon juice
10 oz. cheese, grated, I like sharp
1 lg. tomato, chopped, or more if desired
2 or 3 green onions, chopped
black olives, sliced or chopped
Mix or blend together refried beans and bean dip. Spread in the bottom of a 9-inch x 12-inch glass dish. Then mix together sour cream, mayonnaise, and Picante sauce Spread over the beans. Next, mix avocado, salt, pepper, and lemon juice and spread over sour cream layer. Then sprinkle grated cheese over the avocados. Layer chopped tomatoes onions and olives. Serve cold with tortilla chips or giant Fritos. From the kitchen of Annie

Dressing Recipe

4 eggs, boiled
1 tsp. sage (added to taste)
Biscuits, cornbread and light bread sufficient for recipe
Chicken broth from cooked chicken
¼ tsp. pepper
1/8 tsp. salt
Crumble biscuits, cornbread and light bread. Pour the broth off the chicken onto the bread mixture. Cut up onions and add with eggs and sage and stir in black pepper and a little salt.
From the kitchen of Linda A.

The people who make a difference in your life are not the ones with the most credentials, the most money, or the most awards. They are the ones that care.

Author unknown

Dressing and Turkey Bake

Can Chicken
Can Oysters
Box Soda Crackers
2 Bags Rainbow Bread Crumbs
Dozen Eggs
Onion, Medium, Finely Chopped
½ Stick Celery, Finely Chopped
Carrot, Chopped
Salt And Pepper
Butter
Sage
Broth - Turkey or Chicken
Mix Onion, Celery, Carrot, Salt and Pepper, Sage and Butter. Makes about a cup. Brush Over the Turkey and cook it in a Browning Bag.
From the kitchen of Imodean D.

Texas Style BBQ Sauce

1¼ c. ketchup
⅓ c. brown sugar
⅓ c. Worcestershire Sauce
⅓ c. lemon juice
1 tsp. mustard
Clove garlic
¼ c. butter
Add desired amount jalapenos for heat
Cook on low simmer on stove top for 30 minutes.
From the kitchen of Mildred A.

Marinate Sauce

1 c. Worshershire Sauce
¼ c. soy sauce or lite soy sauce
1 tbsp. smoked hickory
1 tbsp. pepper
1 tbsp. paprika
2 tsp. cumin
2 tsp. garlic powder
½ tsp. onion powder
Salt is optional as the first three ingredients contain a lot of salt.
Stir together ingredients and pour over meat and let set overnight before cooking.
From the kitchen of Carol A.

Jezebel Sauce

8 - 10 oz. apple jelly
8 - 10 oz pineapple preserves
1½ to 2 oz horseradish
2 tbsp. dry mustard
Mix together. Pour over 8 oz. of
cream cheese. Put on Ritz Crackers
From the kitchen of Pat J.

Texas Green Sauce

3 med size green tomatoes, coarsely
    chopped
4 tomatillos (cleaned and chopped)
1 to 2 jalapenos, stemmed, seeded
and coarsely chopped (use gloves)
3 small garlic cloves, chopped
3 medium size ripe avocados - peel
and seed (Ripe avocados are firm
like a tomato but not hard or soft)
4 sprigs cilantro, chopped
1 tsp. salt
1½ c. sour cream
Combine all ingredients and chill.
Serve with Tortilla chips.
From the kitchen of Susanne T.

Hot Sauce

Can whole tomatoes
½ chopped onion
Medium jalapeno, sliced
½ - 1 c. cilantro leaves
Garlic salt
Put all ingredients in blender and
blend. Taste. If too hot, wait a day
to serve.
From the kitchen of Paula H.

Homemade Cheese Whiz

2 tbsp. margarine
1½ lbs. American Processed Cheese
2 egg yolks, beaten
13 oz. can evaporated milk
1 tbsp. flour
In double broiler, melt butter and
add cheese. When softened add egg
yolks, milk and flour. Cook until
thick. Store in a covered dish in the
refrigerator. Hint, use this melted
over cooked macaroni.
From the kitchen of June M.

Peanut Butter Delight Spread

1 c. crunchy peanut butter

1/2 c. unsweetened apple sauce (or small tub of plain Greek Yogurt)

1/3 c. locally produced honey

1 tbsp. extra virgin olive oil

1 tbsp. cinnamon powder

1 tsp. turmeric

Stir well and use on whole grain toast or whole wheat crackers on occasions. Store in the refrigerator.

From the kitchen of Lewis A.

Cheddar Cheese Spread

It's A Volcano!

4 c. (16 oz.) cheddar cheese, shredded

1 tbsp. onion, finely diced

1 c. no fat mayonnaise

1 tsp. hot pepper sauce

1 tsp. pinto bean seasoning

1 tsp Italian seasoning

3 tbsp strawberry jam

1 box wheat crackers

In a bowl, mix cheese, onion, mayonnaise and hot sauce. Spoon the mixture onto a platter or serving dish. Put two plastic sandwich bags or plastic wrap on your hands like gloves, then form the cheese spread into a mound. Form 2 inch x 2 inch hole in the top of the mound. Spoon the jam into the hole. Surround with crackers and add a knife for spreading. Makes a 1 large party spread for twelve people. This can be formed in a ring mold and a small bowl placed in the center to hold the strawberry jam.

From the kitchen of Paul T.

Buttermilk Syrup

1½ c. sugar

¼ c. buttermilk

½ c. butter or margarine

2 tbsp. corn syrup

1 tsp. baking soda

2 tsp. vanilla

In a sauce pan, combine the first five ingredients; bring to a boil. Boil for seven minutes. Remove from the heat; stir in vanilla. .

8 servings, about two cups of syrup.

From the kitchen of Linda A.

Dipping Chocolate

6 oz. chocolate chips
½ bar paraffin
2 Hershey Bars
Melt these items in either top of double boiler or can be done in a microwave oven. It usually takes 2-3 recipes of the dipping chocolate. Cover any type of ball that you create.

Homemade Eagle Brand Milk

1/3 c. boiling water
3 tbsp. melted butter
2/3 c. sugar
1 c. powdered milk
Mix and blend until smooth. This make one can of Eagle Brand Milk.
From the Kitchen of Phyliss T.

Salsa

8 oz can of tomato sauce
14 ½ oz. can of diced tomatoes
2 green onions
1 to 2 fresh seeded jalapenos
2 tbsp. jalapenos and add a couple tbsp of the pickled juice
2 tsp. garlic powder
Small bunch cilantro
salt and pepper to taste

Combine all ingredients in a blender. Blend until well blended. Put in quart jar and put in the refrigerator overnight.
From the kitchen of Debbie W.

South of the Border Pepitas Dip

½ c. pumpkin seeds, toasted
2 Poblano Chiles, roasted, seeded, and peeled
1 clove garlic, peeled
½ tsp. sea salt and ½ c. cilantro
¼ tsp. freshly ground black pepper
½ c. canola oil
2 tbsp. red wine vinegar
¼ c. crumbled goat cheese
½ c. light olive oil mayonnaise
½ c. warm water
carrots and celery, cut in strips
Place seed, chilies, garlic, salt, pepper, oil, vinegar, cheese and cilantro. Puree to a smooth consistency. Add mayo and enough warm water to create your desired consistency. Place in the fridge to allow to blend and thicken. Serve with crudités.
From the kitchen of Chef Nancy W

Chapter 5
Soup and Chowder

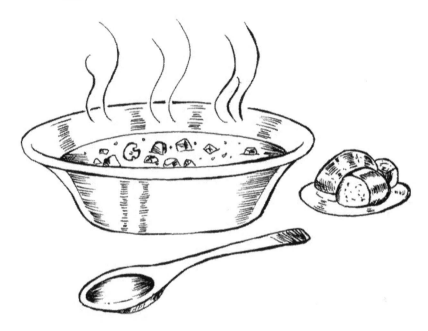

Index of Soup and Chowder Recipes

Santa Fe Chicken Soup

(Hearty Soup)

½ to ¾ stick margarine
Sauté: 1 large onion sliced
Sauté: 4 chicken breast, cut in 1" cubes (about 1½ lbs of chicken)
4 oz. can diced green chilies
3 cloves garlic, minced
1 can Swanson chicken broth
3 or 4 cubes chicken bouillon (4 tsp.)
4 c. boiling water
1½ lbs. fresh Roma tomatoes, chopped very course or 2 cans tomatoes
2 or 3 bay leaves
Italian seasoning (1 tsp. or to taste)
Fresh mushrooms or 1 can mushroom caps
½ to 1 c. diced carrots
1 c. celery, chopped
Throw into a pot and simmer 1 - 1½ hours. Serve with Tostado chips or crackers.
From the kitchen of Bruce H.

Taco Soup

Combine:
2 lbs. ground beef
Onion, chopped
Mix in dry seasonings:
Pkg. taco seasoning
Pkg. Hidden Valley Ranch Seasoning
Brown beef and onion together.
Garlic powder to taste
Can whole tomatoes: puree
Can yellow corn, drained
Can Rotel tomatoes
Can pinto beans, rinsed
Can kidney beans, rinsed
Add beef mixture. Simmer together 30 minutes. Serve over tortilla chips and top with shredded cheese.
From the kitchen of Alecia M.

Do you know why a car's WINDSHIELD is so large and the rear view mirror is so small? Because our PAST is not as important as our FUTURE. So, look ahead and move on.

Chicken Barley Chili

14.5 oz. can tomatoes, diced, undrained

16 oz. jar/can salsa or tomato sauce

14.5 oz. fat free chicken broth

1 c. Quaker Quick Barley

3 c. water

1 tbsp. chili powder

1 tsp. cumin

15 oz. can black beans, drained and rinsed.

15 oz. corn, whole kennel or with peppers, undrained.

3 c. chicken breast, (1 ½ lb) cooked, cut into bite-sized pieces (canned chicken may be used.)

Optional:

Reduced or no fat cheddar cheese

Reduced fat or fat free sour cream

In 6 quart saucepan, combine the first 7 ingredients. Over high heat bring to a boil; cover and reduce heat to low. Simmer for 20 minutes, stirring occasionally. Add beans, corn and chicken; increase heat to high until chili comes to a boil. Cover and reduce heat to low. Simmer for another five minutes, or until the barley is tender. If upon standing the chili becomes too thick, add some more chicken broth or water until chili is desired consistency. (If desired, top with shredded cheese and sour cream.) Makes 11 - one cup servings. From the Barley box, an Emporia State Christian Student Center favorite. From the kitchen of Linda A.

King Ranch Chicken Soup

3-4 chicken breasts

Medium onion, chopped

Can Rotel tomatoes

Can cream of chicken soup,

Can or 2 cans fresh or frozen corn

salt and pepper and garlic

1 lb. Velveeta cheese

Cornmeal

Flour

Milk

Cover chicken breasts with water, simmer until cooked. Remove and cut up into bite size pieces. Return to broth. Add next 6 ingredients to the chicken and broth. Simmer for 30 minutes. Add Veletta cheese. Thicken with cornmeal, flour and milk. Serve. From the kitchen of Paula H.

Vegetable Barley Soup

½ lb. lean ground beef
½ c. chopped onion
1 clove garlic, minced
5 c. water
14½ oz. can unsalted whole tomatoes, undrained, cut into pieces
¾ c. Quick Quaker Barley
½ c. sliced celery
½ c. sliced carrots
2 beef bouillon cubes
½ tsp. dried basil, crushed
1 bay leaf
9 oz. pkg. frozen mixed vegetables

In a 4-quart saucepan or Dutch oven, brown meat. Add onion and garlic; cook until onion is tender. Drain. Stir in remaining ingredients except frozen vegetable. Cover, bring to a boil. Reduce heat; simmer 10 minutes, stirring occasionally. Add frozen vegetables; cook about 10 minutes or until vegetables are tender. Additional water may be added if soup becomes too thick upon standing. Makes 8 one cup servings. From the Quaker Barley box. This was a favorite at the ESU Christian Student Center at Emporia, Kansas on Fridays. From the kitchen of Linda A.

Grating Cheese

Love using hard cheeses as opposed to the shredded stuff in the store. Do you always nick your finger tips when grating cheese. So, cover two or three of your fingers with metal thimbles. Now, you can grate much faster and closer.

Quick Asparagus Soup

Can asparagus spears (whole or cut)
Can chicken broth
Salt and pepper (white) to taste
Fresh parsley, minced

In a blender, puree the asparagus shears with their liquid and add chicken broth. Heat, adding salt and pepper to taste. Sprinkle with parsley, serve hot. Great as an appetizer. Serve in small cups before the meal.
From the kitchen of Barbara C.

Southwest Taco Chili Soup

1 lb. Lean Ground Sirloin Beef, cooked and drained. (Melba used ground round.)
1 med. red onion, chopped
1 tbsp. minced garlic
2 c. chicken stock (not broth)
1.5 oz. package Nueva Concina Taco Fresco Seasoning
15 oz. can Hunt's Roasted Diced Tomatoes with Garlic
14 oz. can Rotel Mild Diced Tomatoes
2 cans Green Giant Mexicorn
15 oz. can Bush's Black Beans
15 oz. can Ranch Style Beans
(Optional: grated cheese and sour cream)

In a large pot over medium heat, add onions and beef; brown until cooked through. Stir in seasonings and broth and the rest of the ingredients. Simmer for 20 minutes or until all is hot. Place in bowls and cover with crushed tortilla chips.

From the kitchen of Melba R.

Chicken Tortilla Soup

1½ lbs boneless chicken, cooked and shredded
Can (15 oz.) whole tomatoes
Can (10 oz.) enchilada sauce
Medium onion, chopped
Can (4 oz.) green chilies, chopped
Clove garlic, minced
2 c. water
Can (14½ oz.) chicken broth
1 tsp. cumin
1 tsp. chili powder and 1 tsp. salt
¼ tsp. black pepper
1 bay leaf
Pkg. (10 oz.) frozen corn
1 tbsp. dried cilantro, chopped
6 corn tortillas
2 tbsp. vegetable oil
Parmesan cheese, grated, for garnish

In crock-pot, combine the shredded chicken, tomatoes, enchilada sauce, onion, green chilies, and garlic. Add water, chicken broth, cumin, chili powder, salt, black pepper, and bay leaf. Stir in the corn and cilantro. Cover and cook on LO 6 - 8 hours or on HI 3 - 4 hours.

Preheat oven to 400° F. Lightly brush both sides of tortillas with vegetable oil. Cut the tortillas into strips that are 2½ inches long and ½ inch wide. Spread the tortilla strips onto a baking sheet. Bake, turning occasionally.

From the kitchen of Catherine G.

Paula's Original Tortilla Soup

4 chicken breasts
1 can Rotel tomatoes
½ c. chopped onion
1 tsp. cumin
½ tsp. garlic powder
Salt and pepper
Can ranch style beans undrained
    shredded cheddar cheese
Cilantro sprigs

Boil chicken breasts covered in water until tender. Remove chicken, de-bone and cut into bite size pieces. Return to chicken broth in the cooking pot. Add the tomatoes, onion, cumin, garlic powder, and beans. Season with salt and pepper as desired. Cook until the onion is tender, about 30 minutes. Serve topped with shredded cheese and with cilantro if desired.

From the kitchen of Paula H.

Ham Chowder

¼ c. butter
1 c. onion, chopped
1 c. celery, chopped
2 c. diced potatoes
2 c. diced ham
2 c. water
1 bay leaf
¾ tsp. salt
Dash pepper
1/3 tsp. thyme
½ c. milk

Melt butter in pot. Add onions and celery. Cook until translucent. Add bay leaf and spices. Add potatoes and ham. Cover with two cups of water, cook until potatoes are soft. Add milk and serve hot. (Better if served with sweet cornbread)

From the kitchen of Tim T.

Cream of Bacon Swiss Mushroom Soup

Can of cream of mushroom soup
Can of water
3 slices of aged Swiss cheese
Mix soup and water and heat. Cut up cheese and add then heat until melted. Cook 4 slices of crisp bacon and crumble over the top of the soup and serve.
From the kitchen of Alex B.

Cheese Broccoli Soup

½ gal. 2% milk
2 tbsp. dried parsley
1/8 lb. mild cheddar cheese
½ large brick Velveeta cheese
½ lb. butter
flour
1 onion
2 bunches fresh broccoli
1½ tsp. instant chicken bouillon
½ tsp. garlic salt
dash of pepper
Make a Rue. Over med heat, melt ½ lb. butter. Add flour until almost too thick to stir. Make sure there are no lumps. Consider using a hand mixer if help is needed. Finely chop and clean fresh broccoli and onions. Put two inches of water in large pan and add broccoli, onions, bouillon, parsley, pepper, and garlic salt. Bring to boil and simmer about 20 minutes. Add milk (do not boil) and Rue until creamy. About 30 minutes prior to serving slowly add cheeses, cubed into small pieces. Makes about ¾ gallon.
From the kitchen of Catherine G.

Corn Chowder

Cook:
3 slices of bacon in microwave
  and crumble
Sauté:
¼ c. onion, chopped, add small amount of olive or canola oil to sauté onions in stock pot
Add to Stock Pot:
crumbled bacon and onion
2 c. cream style corn (1 can)
2 c. finely diced, raw potato
1 c. finely cut celery
1 c. finely cut carrots
1 c. boiling water over the
  potatoes
Cook until potatoes, celery, and carrots are tender (10-15 minutes)
Stir often.

Just before serving, add:

2+ c. milk (evaporated, skim or whole milk)

Season to Taste:

½ - 1 tsp. salt

1/8 tsp. pepper

Heat to simmering, stirring occasionally. Serve immediately. Serves about six. This recipe can be doubled or tripled.

From the kitchen of Linda A.

Potato Soup with Dumplings

Soup:

1 c. celery, diced

½ c. water

6 med. potatoes, chopped in small pieces

2 tsp. salt

¼ tsp. pepper

3 c. milk

Dumplings:

1 c. flour, sifted

½ tsp. salt

½ tsp. sugar

1 tsp. parsley

1 egg

½ c. milk

Stir together the dumpling ingredients and roll into a log. Slice into small chunks. Mix the soup ingredients and bring to a slow boil and then drop in the dumpling chunks, and boil for addition 20 minutes.

From the kitchen of Ethel A.

Recipe for Happiness

4 cups of love

2 cups of loyalty

3 cups of kindness

1 cup of friendship

5 spoons of hope

5 spoons of faith

1 barrel of laughter

Take love and loyalty and mix thoroughly with faith.

Blend it with:

Tenderness, kindness, understanding, and forgiveness.

Add hope and friendship.

Sprinkle abundantly with laughter.

Bake with sunshine.

Serve daily with generous helpings.

Author Unknown

Chapter 6
Fruit and Fruit Salad

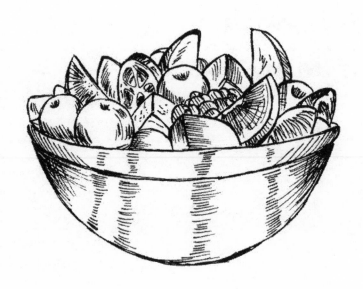

Index of Fruit and Fruit Salad Recipes

Mother's Strawberry Jello Salad

Pkg. strawberry jello

1 c. boiling water

Pkg. cream cheese

Sm. can crushed pineapple with juice

Pkg. frozen strawberries

Dissolve jello in boiling water. Cut up package of package of cream cheese, add to hot jello and blend together in blender. Pour into serving bowls. Stir in strawberries and pineapple.

From the kitchen of Irene T.

Mandarin Orange Salad

lg. box orange jello

lg. cool whip

8 oz. sour cream

2 - 8 oz. cans Mandarin oranges

Small can crushed pineapple

1 c. chopped pecans

Blend cool whip and sour cream. Add jello and blend well. Stir in oranges, pineapple and pecans.

Chill in refrigerator.

From the kitchen of Linda A.

Mandarin Orange Salad

Dressing:

¼ c. olive oil

4 tsp. balsamic vinegar or more

1½ tsp. Dijon style mustard

¼ tsp. salt and ¼ tsp. pepper

Combine the vinegar, mustard, salt and pepper in a small bowl. Stir together until blended.

Salad:

Pkg. baby spinach or other salad blend

Can (11 oz. or 15 oz.) Mandarin oranges, drained.

2 tbsp. sliced ripe olives

½ c. red onion, sliced

¼ c. feta cheese, crumbled

Stir together spinach, mandarin oranges, olives and onion in a large serving bowl. Pour dressing over the salad; toss evenly to coat. Top with feta cheese. Recipe makes 4 servings.

From the kitchen of Debbie W.

Mother's Lime Jello Salad

Small box of lime Jello
1 c. boiling water
1 c. small marsh mellows or 8 large
6 oz. cream cheese.
10 ice cubes
Small can pineapple, crushed
½ c. nuts
Dissolve jello in cup of boiling water. Add marsh mellows and cream cheese. Use blender to blend above ingredients. Stir in ice cubes. Stir in the pineapple and nuts. After it starts to thicken, remove any ice cubes that remain and stir.
Refrigerate until set and ready to serve.
From the kitchen of Irene T.

Jello Salad

1 lg. or 2 sm. pkg. orange jello
2 c. boiling water
Small can frozen orange juice
1 c. cold water
Can drained mandarin oranges
6 oz. miniature marsh-mellows
Small box instant lemon pudding
9 oz. cartoon Cool Whip
Dissolve jello in boiling water. Add orange juice, cold water and oranges. Layer with marsh mellows. Cool until jello is set. Layer with pudding mixed according to directions on box. Top with Cool Whip.
From the kitchen of Catherine G.

Fruit Bowl

2 cans Mandarin oranges
2 cans chunk pineapple
Small pkg. strawberries (thawed)
Can peach pie filling
4 bananas (Sprinkle with fruit fresh to keep from browning.)
Drain liquid off and mix all ingredients except bananas.
Prepare night before serving. Just before serving, cut up the bananas and add.
From the kitchen of June M.

Fruit Salad and Dressing

1 c. pineapple juice

1 egg

1 c. sugar

Juice of 1 lemon

3 tsp. flour

Dash of salt

Mix and cook on low flame until thick. Stir constantly. Set in refrigerator to cool.

Pour over:

1 c. pineapple chunks

1 c. grapes

2 oranges, peeled and sectioned

1 apple cut into pieces

½ c. nuts coarsely chopped

1 c. marshmallows

3 bananas, sliced

From the kitchen of Pat J.

White Chocolate Fruit Salad

2 - 8 oz. cool whip

2 - 8 oz. sour cream

2 - sm. white chocolate instant pudding

Can medium crushed pineapple (drained)

2 cans fruit cocktail (drained)

Mix cool whip and sour cream together, mix in pudding a little at a time, then add fruit.

Refrigerate.

From the kitchen of Debbie W.

White Chocolate Ambrosia

15 oz. can lite fruit cocktail

20 oz. can pineapple tidbits in its own juice

11 oz. can mandarin oranges

½ c. drained, sliced cherries (optional)

2 small pkg. fat free white chocolate instant pudding mix

1 c. fat free sour cream

½ - 12 oz. tub fat free Cool Whip

Drain fruits, but retain 1½ cup of liquid.(any lite syrup - toss and replace with a true fruit juice.) In large bowl whisk juice with pudding mix until it thickens. Stir in sour cream and Cool Whip. Fold in fruits and chill. Chopped pecans can be added. Recipe can easily be doubled or tripled and is better on the day after it is prepared. Serves 10-12. Can add the other ½ of the tub if desired. From the kitchen of Bobbye P.

Baked Apple Connecticut

4 baking apples, cored
Lemon juice
¾ c. sugar
¼ tsp. nutmeg
2 tbsp. butter or margarine
¼ c. water
Dip cut ends of apples in lemon juice. Place in a baking dish. Fill centers of apples with sugar mixture. Dot apple tops with butter. Pour water into bottom of baking dish. Cover. Bake in a moderate oven (350° F.) for 1¼ hours.
From unknown kitchen

Cheesecake and Fruit Dessert Pizza

Pkg. (16 oz.) Refrigerated sugar cookie dough
12 oz. cream cheese, softened
¼ c. sugar
Can (11 or 15 oz. Mandarin oranges
2 kiwi fruit, peeled, sliced
¾ c. strawberries
½ c. raspberries (optional)
Press cookie dough on bottom of lightly greased 12 inch pizza pan. Bake at 350° F. or until light brown. Cool to room temperature. Beat cream cheese and sugar in medium bowl until smooth and blended. Stir in ½ cup mandarin oranges. Spread over crust. Cover and refrigerate until ready to serve. Arrange kiwi, strawberries, raspberries and remaining mandarin oranges over cream cheese before serving. Garnish with mint leaves, if desired. Makes 12 servings.
From the kitchen of Linda A.

Pineapple -Walnut Dessert

Pkg. (7½ oz.) vanilla wafers
1 c. butter or margarine
1 c. sugar
2 tsp. vanilla
2 eggs
2 c. well drained crushed
    pineapple
1 c. walnuts, finely chopped

Crush vanilla wafers to fine crumbs, reserve 2 tbsp. Cream butter and add sugar gradually add vanilla. Add eggs, one at a time, beating well. Combine pineapple and walnuts, stirring in until well mixed. Line a 8 inch x 5 inch x 3 inch loaf pan with foil, leaving overhanging so loaf can be easily lifted out. Press ½ cup crumbs on the bottom of the pan. Add about ¼ pineapple mixture, spreading evenly. Repeat until crumbs and pineapple mixture used up, ending with the latter. Scatter reserved crumbs on top. Chill 24 hours or longer before serving (or freeze.) Garnish with whipped cream and Maraschino cherries, if desired. Slice to serve. Serves 10-12

Hawaiian Dessert

Pkg. 18¼ ounces yellow cake
    mix
3 pkg. (3.4 oz. each) instant vanilla
    pudding mix
4 c. cold milk
1½ tsp. coconut extract
Pkg. (8 oz.) cream cheese,
    softened
Can (20 oz.) crushed pineapple
    well drained
2 c. heavy cream, whipped and
    sweetened
2 c. flaked coconut, toasted

Mix cake batter according to pkg. directions.
Pour into two, greased 13 inch x 9 inch baking pan. Bake at 350° F. for 15 minutes or until the cake test done. Cool completely. In large mixing bowl, combine pudding mixes and milk in a bowl. Spread on the baked cakes.   Add whipped cream on top of the cakes and sprinkle with toasted coconut.   Chill for at least two hours. (Prepared dessert can be covered and frozen for up to one month.)
From the kitchen of Phyllis T.

Geraldine's Cherry Pudding

Can cherries
Pkg. cherry jello
1 c. sugar (May use brown sugar)
4 eggs
36 Vanilla wafers or a few more
 ½ c. or more nuts

Place in sauce pan cherry juice from can and enough water to make a cup of liquid, to this add sugar and beat egg yolks and add to mixture and cook slowly until it thickens or eggs are 'cooked' (a short time) Beat egg whites and pour mixture from sauce pan into the whites and mix. Pour in flat pan or leave in bowl and serve plain or with whipped cream. Chill.

From the kitchen of Andrea B.

Remember the Five Simple Rules to Be Happy

1. Free your heart from hatred.
2. Free your mind from worries.
3. Live simply.
4. Give more.
5. Expect less.

Better than Momma's Banana Pudding

Vanilla wafers
4-6 bananas
2 c. milk
5 oz. instant French vanilla
 pudding
8 oz. cream cheese
14 oz. sweetened condensed milk
12 oz. frozen whipped topping,
 thawed

Line the bottom of a 13-inch x 9-inch dish with vanilla wafers, layer sliced bananas on top. In a bowl combine milk and pudding in mixer, in another bowl combine cream cheese and condensed milk together, mix until smooth. Fold the whipped topping into the cream cheese mixture and stir until well blended. Pour the mixture over cookies and bananas and cover with cookies.
Refrigerate until ready to serve.
From unknown kitchen

Date Pudding

2 c. chopped dates
1 c. boiling water
2 tbsp. of oil or margarine
1 c. sugar
1 tsp. vanilla
1½ c. flour
1 tsp. soda and 1 tsp. baking
    powder
½ tsp. salt
2/3 c. nut meats, chopped
1 egg
Stir in dates and water, let stand 5 minutes, cream fat and sugar and add. Stir in the rest of the ingredients. Pour into a greased and floured pan 13-inch x 9-inch x 2-inch. Bake 40 minutes at 350° F, then serve plain or top with whipped cream. Serves 12-15.
From the kitchen of Maxine K.

Pantry Pudding Surprise

4 c. corn flakes, crushed
⅓ c. brown sugar, firmly packed
½ tsp. cinnamon
⅓ margarine, melted
Pkg. vanilla instant pudding mix
    made as directed.

Combine 3½ cup cereal, sugar, and margarine. Set aside. Press ½ cup mixture into the bottom of 8-inch pan. Pour pudding over cereal mixture. Top with remaining ½ cup cereal. Chill for an hour.
From Unknown kitchen.

Lemon Cloud

2 sticks margarine
2 c. flour
2 c. confectioners' sugar
2 (8oz.) pkg. cream cheese
2 boxes lemon instant pudding
3 c. milk
Large container of Cool Whip
Mix margarine and flour together for crust. Press into a 9 inch x 13 inch pan. Bake at 350° F. for 20 - 25 minutes. Cool. Whip confectioners' sugar and cream cheese and put on crust. Mix lemon pudding and milk. Put on top. Spread Cool Whip on top. Refrigerate.
From the kitchen of June T.

Never give the devil a ride -- he will always want to drive.

58

Cool Whip Salad

Jar Marchino cherries, cut in half
Large carton Cool Whip
2 large bananas, mashed
½ c. nuts
Can crushed pineapple, drained
2 tbsp. fresh lemon juice
2 - 4 tbsp. sugar
Mash bananas. Add sugar and lemon juice. Mix well. Fold into the Cool Whip with remaining ingredients. May be served immediately or refrigerate for later in the day. Otherwise freeze and cut into squares.
From the kitchen of Phyliss T.

"I believe that we don't have to change friends if we understand that friends change."

Keep an open mind. Discuss but don't argue. It is a mark of a superior mind to be able to disagree without being disagreeable.

Pear Honey

4 c. pears, peeled, crushed
3 c. sugar
¼ tsp. salt
Lemon, ground
Combine all ingredients and cook in a heavy pan, stirring occasionally for about 15 minutes or until spreading consistency. Pour into hot jars. Adjust lids at once and process in boiling water bath (212° F.) 5 minutes. Remove from canner and complete seals unless closers are self sealing type. It makes 2½ pints. For variation: Orange/Pear Honey - use orange instead of lemon.
From the kitchen of Irene A.

All things in life are temporary. If it's going well, enjoy it, they will not last forever. If it's going wrong, don't worry, they can't last long either.

Chapter 7
Vegetables and Salads

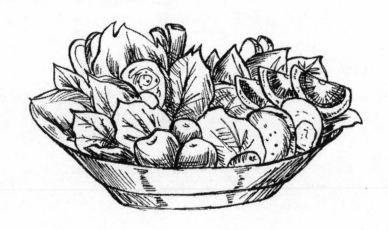

Index of Vegetable and Salad Recipes

German Potato Salad

6 c. hot diced potatoes
1/3 c. finely chopped onions
9 slices bacon, cooked crisp, crumbled
3 tbsp. bacon drippings
¾ c. vinegar
1 tbsp. sugar
¾ c. boiling water
1½ tbsp. prepared mustard
1 c. dairy sour cream
1 tbsp. finely chopped parsley
Mix all ingredients and then salt and pepper to taste.
From the kitchen of Catherine G.

Greek Potato Salad

6 new red potatoes
Goodly portion of parsley
Bunch of green onions
Bunch of celery
Large clove of garlic
1 tsp. salt
1 tsp. pepper
2 tbsp. paprika
Juice of one lemon
½ c. olive oil
½ c salad oil
½ c. juice of dill pickles
¼ c. vinegar

Boil the potatoes with skins and allow to cool. Very finely chop and mix a good portion of parsley, onions and celery. Set aside. Create sauce by first mashing or pressing one large clove of garlic. Add each of the remaining ingredients. Taste for tartness. Peel potatoes and cut in thin slices. Layer potatoes, green ingredients, ending with sauce. Cover and refrigerate for several hours.
From the kitchen of Phyliss T.

My Wish for You

May the pockets of your jeans become a magnet for $100 bills.
May love stick to your face like Vaseline and may laughter assault your lips!
May happiness slap you across the face and may your tears be that of joy
May the problems you had, forget your home address!
In simple words, may each successive year be the best year of Your Life.

Gussie's Potato Salad

3 lb. boiled potatoes
8 boiled eggs
Medium onion, chopped
1 c. minced sweet pickles
1 c. mayonnaise
½ c. pickle juice and milk
1½ tbsp. mustard
2 tbsp. sugar
1½ tsp. celery seed
¼ tsp. pepper
1 tsp. salt - optional
In a large bowl, mash or cut into chunks the potatoes. Add the eggs, onion, and pickles. Combine rest of the ingredients in a bowl and add to potato mix. Taste. May need to add more pickle juice or milk.
From the Kitchen of Linda A.

Quick Scalloped Potatoes

6 med. potatoes (about 6 oz. each)
¼ c. butter or margarine
1 tbsp. dried onion flakes
1 tsp. salt
½ tsp. pepper
¼ c. flour
2 c. milk

Stir together in a microwave dish, cover, then cook for 10 minutes on high. Serve.
From the kitchen of Mildred A.

Scalloped Potatoes

6-8 medium potatoes
Can mushroom soup
1 c. milk
1 tsp. salt
1 chopped onion
Pepper as desired
Mix the milk and salt in with the soup, onion and pepper and pour over the sliced potatoes. Bake 1½ hours at a low temperature.
From the kitchen of Melba R.

Hash Brown Casserole

2 lb. bag of frozen hash brown potatoes
¼ c. chopped onion
Can cream of chicken soup
1 pt. of sour cream
2 c. of grated cheese (Mild Cheddar)
1 tsp. salt
½ tsp. pepper
Mix: all these ingredients together and pour in a greased 9-inch x 13-inch Pyrex pan.
Topping:
2 c. of crushed potato chips or corn lakes
½ c. of melted margarine.
Pour the melted margarine over the crushed chips/flakes and spread that over the top of the casserole. Bake at 350° F. for 45 minutes.
From the kitchen of Suzanne T.

Hash Brown Potato Bake

½ c. onion
¼ c. oleo
Pkg. (2 lb.) frozen hash brown potatoes
Can cream of celery soup
Carton sour cream
½ c. milk
1 tsp. salt
½ tsp. pepper
Sauté onions with oleo. Mix in other ingredients and pour over hash brown potatoes in large baking dish. Sprinkle 1½ cups grated Velveeta cheese over the potato mixture. Top with 2 cups crushed potato chips mixed with ¼ cup melted oleo. Bake at 450° F. for 45 minutes.
From the kitchen of Phyliss T.

Sweet Potato Bake

2 sweet potatoes and ¼ c. sugar
⅓ c. butter and 1 tsp. vanilla
Slice the potatoes and lay then in a casserole disk Mix together the sugar, butter and vanilla and spread over the potatoes.
Top with a mixture of:
¼ c. brown sugar
¼ c. butter with cinnamon and pecans as desired. Bake at 350° F. for 35 minutes.
From the kitchen of Imodean D.

Sweet Potato Casserole

4 or 5 med. sweet potatoes
Stick butter
2 eggs
1 c. coconut
1 c. sugar
1 tsp. vanilla
1 tsp. salt

Topping:
1 c. chopped pecans
¾ stick of butter, melted
1 c. flour
Mix together and put on top of potatoes. Bake in 9 inch x 13 inch dish at 350° F. for 30-45 minutes or until well.
From the kitchen of Alecia M.

Pineapple Marshmellow Sweet Potato

2 c. sweet potatoes, mashed
1 c. milk
½ c. pineapple juice
2 tbsp. butter
½ tsp. cinnamon
marsh-mellows
Thoroughly mix all ingredients, beat until light and fluffy. Use more milk or fruit juice if needed. Place in a buttered casserole dish and bake until heated throughout. Remove from oven and cover the top with marshmallows. Return to oven to brown. Serve with poultry or roast.
From the kitchen of Ethel A.

Vegetable Pie

Crust:
½ c. butter
1¼ c. whole wheat flour
2 tsp. baking powder
½ tsp. salt
½ c. plain yogurt

Filling:
2 c. broccoli, finely chopped
½ c. onion, diced
1 c. grated cheese
2 med. tomatoes, sliced
1/3 c. mayo
1 tsp. basil
Cut butter into flour, baking powder and salt. Add yogurt. Pat the dough into greased 9 inch or 10 inch pie pan. Layer filling over crust in order given. Bake at 450° F. for 10 minutes; then at 350° F. for another ½ hour.
From the kitchen of Janet K.

Texas Panhandle Cabbage Salad

Large head Chinese cabbage
Large bell pepper
6-8 green onions
2 pkg. Ramon Noodle Mix chicken
    flavor or oriental
¾ c. almonds, sliced or slivered and
    ½ c. sesame seeds
2 tbsp. oleo
1/3 c. rice wine vinegar
2/3 c. sugar
1 tsp. pepper
2 tsp. salt
1 c. salad oil
Chop the cabbage, pepper and onions, and seal in a zip loc bag Combine the almonds, and sesame seeds and toast in oleo. Heat to boiling the wine vinegar and add sugar, pepper, and salt. Mix in the flavoring and seeds. Allow to cool then add salad oil. When ready to serve, mix salad and noodles. Shake salad dressing and pour over the salad and serve.
From the kitchen of Ida U.

Baked Shredded Carrots

3 tbsp. butter or oleo
⅓ c. onions, finely chopped
1½ c. carrots, shredded
¾ c. water
1½ tsp. lemon juice
¾ tsp. ginger
1½ tbsp. sugar
1 tsp. salt
3 more tbsp. butter or oleo
Heat oven to 350° F. Melt first 3 tablespoons of butter or oleo in skillet, add onions and cook over moderate heat until tender. Add carrots and pour into a 2 quart casserole dish. Mix water, lemon juice, ginger, and salt. Pour over carrots. Dot with 3 tablespoons of butter or oleo. Cover and bake for 60 minutes or until tender.
From the kitchen of Ethel A.

Black Eyed Pea Salad

4 cans black eyed peas, drained
Can jalapeño black eyed peas
½ c. chopped purple onion
½ c. diced green pepper
Can Rotel tomatoes, undrained
1 tsp. sugar
Small bottle Italian dressing
4 ripe but firm avocadoes
salt and pepper to taste
From the kitchen of Phyllis T.

Chick Pea Stuffed Acorn Squash

2 acorn squash, halved and seeds
   removed
½ c. canned chick peas, drained
1 tbsp. olive oil
2 stalk celery, chopped
Carrot, grated
1/8 c. tamari
1 tbsp. parsley
½ tsp. ground cumin
Clove garlic, crushed
¼ tsp. salt
1/8 tsp. turmeric
3 tbsp. Tahiti or peanut butter
Prick squash skins, bake at 350° F.
for 45 minutes or until soft, or
microwave on HI for 20 minutes.
Mash chick peas. Sauté garlic and
onion in oil until soft. Add celery,
carrot, tamari and seasonings. Stir 5
minutes more. Remove from heat.
Add chick peas and mix. Add
remaining ingredients except squash.
Stuff acorns and bake at 375° F. for
25 minutes.
From the kitchen of Janet K.

English Pea and Corn Salad

16 oz. can English peas, drain well
Can shoe peg corn, drain well
1 c. green bell pepper, chopped and
1 c. celery, diced
4 or 5 green onions, chopped - use
   some tops
Small jar diced pimiento
DRESSING
½ c. sugar
½ c. vinegar
½ c. oil
½ tsp. salt
Stir together to dissolve sugar.

Catherine's Beans

8 slices of bacon

4 med onions, chopped

Can (#1) green beans, drained

Can (#1) lima beans, drained

Can (14 oz.) pork and beans

Can (#1) kidney beans, undrained

¾ c. dark brown sugar

½ c. vinegar

½ tsp. garlic salt

½ tsp. dry mustard

Pepper to taste

Fry bacon crisp. Save bacon drippings. Drain and crumble. Sauté onions in bacon drippings until transparent. Thoroughly drain onions. Combine all beans, onion and bacon. Combine brown sugar, vinegar, garlic salt, mustard and pepper and add to the beans. Mix well. Bake uncovered in 3 quart casserole at 350° F. for 1 hour. Freezes nicely. Serves 16.

From the kitchen of Irene T.

Friendship is like a BOOK. It takes few seconds to burn, but it takes years to write.

Ruby's Bean Salad

1 c. fresh beans

1 c. English peas

4 sticks celery, chopped

Small can pimentos

Small can Vienna sausage

Medium onion, cut finely

¼ c. Wesson Oil

¾ sugar

1 tsp. salt

½ c. white vinegar

Mix well. Toss vegetable, pour liquids over salad. Set for one hour and drain.

From the kitchen of Ruby K.

Squash Dish

2 tbsp. olive oil

¼ c. chopped onion

Zucchini squash, sliced

Yellow squash, sliced

Can Delmonte Dice Tomatoes in basil, oregano and garlic

Cook the onions in the olive oil until they are tender. Then add the squash and cook until slightly tender. Add the tomatoes, cover and simmer until cooked about 20 minutes plus.

From the kitchen of Melba R.

Sonora Casserole

	Big Feast	Small Feast
Sliced zucchini	3 lbs.	1½ lbs.
Frozen corn	½ lb.	¼ lb.
Tortilla Chips	4 lbs.	2 lbs.
Diced green chili	5 oz.	2½ oz.
Vinegar	1 tsp.	½ tsp.
Paprika	1 tsp.	½ tsp.
Cumin	1 tsp.	½ tsp.
Shredded cheese	2 lbs.	1 lb.
Tomato sauce	32 oz.	16 oz.

Cook zucchini. Mix other ingredients together. Add zucchini. Bake at 350°F. for 30 minutes. Layer chips zucchini (barely cooked, corn. Mix chilies, seasoning in tomato sauce and pour over chips and zucchini. Top with cheese. From the kitchen of the 410 Diner, on Broadway, San Antonio.

Zucchini Pie

4 c. sliced or diced zucchini

1 c. chopped onion

¼ to ½ c. butter, olive or Canola oil

½ c. chopped parsley or 2 tbsp. parsley flakes

½ tsp. salt and ½ tsp. pepper

¼ tsp. garlic powder

¼ tsp. basil

¼ tsp. oregano (or more)

2 eggs

8 oz. shredded mozzarella cheese

8 oz. pkg. crescent rolls

2 tbsp. Dijon mustard

Cook zucchini and onions uncovered in butter or oil, until tender - about 10 minutes. Stir in seasonings. In large bowl blend eggs and cheese. Stir in vegetable mixture. Unroll crescent rolls and place dough in an un-greased 12-inch x 8-inch baking dish, press to form crust. Spread mustard over dough evenly. Pour in vegetable mixture. Bake 375° F. for 20 minutes until set. Let stand 10 minutes and serve.

From the kitchen of Sue M.

Zucchini Butter

4 c. zucchini puree
2 c. tart apples, puree
4 tbsp. vinegar
1 tsp. lemon juice
2 c. sugar
2 tsp. cinnamon
Dash of allspice

Peal, seed zucchini and chop. Put zucchini in a blender with vinegar and blend until smooth. Pour in saucepan with remaining ingredients and cook, stirring occasionally until mixture reaches desired thickness. Cool and keep in the refrigerator until ready to serve. Tastes like apple butter.

From the kitchen of Imodean D.

Zucchini Jam

6 c. peeled, grated zucchini
6 c. sugar
2 tbsp. lemon
Can (20 oz) crushed pineapple, well
    drained
2 pkg. (3 oz.) apricot gelatin

Add 1 cup water to zucchini, bring to a boil and cook for 6 minutes. Add gelatin and cook for 6 more minutes. Seal in jelly glasses or pint jars.

From the kitchen of Imodean D.

Be cheerful. Don't burden or depress those around you by dwelling on your aches and pains and small disappointments. Remember, everyone is carrying some kind of burden.

Author unknown

Okra Salad

6 slices bacon, fried crisp, crumbled
Bunch green onions, diced
½ bell pepper, diced
2 tomatoes, seeded and chopped
Medium bag breaded okra, or fixed like mother prepared okra to cook.

Fry okra, cool - mix okra, tomatoes, green onion, bell pepper and bacon. Mix together as a dressing

¼ c. oil
¼ c. sugar
1/8 c. vinegar

Just before serving, pour the dressing over the salad.

From the kitchen of Phyliss T.

Microwave Steamed Okra

Choose fresh, tender, small okra
   pods
Wash. Do not cut off stems.
Arrange in a glass pie plate with the
pod stems to the outside and the
pointed ends toward the center of
the plate. Add ½ tablespoon of
water. Cover with wax paper.
Microwave HI for 2 - 2½ minutes.
Should be tender crisp. Do not
overcook. Adjust the time and
water to the amount of okra you are
steaming. These may be served as a
finger food by picking up the pod
stems.
From the kitchen of Linda A.

Liz's Slaw

2 heads of cabbage, shredded
Vidalia onion or purple onion,
   chopped
1 lb. bacon, fried crisp, crumbled
green and red pepper, chopped fine.
Whisk Wishbone Italian dressings
with bacon drippings. Mix the

chopped and shredded vegetables
and pour the dressing over vegetable
mixture.
From the kitchen of Elizabeth B.

There are moments in life when you
miss someone so much that you just
want to pick them from your
dreams and hug them for real!

24 Hour Cole Slaw

7/8 c. sugar
1 c. vinegar
¾ c. salad oil
2 tbsp. sugar
1 tbsp. salt
1 tsp. dry mustard
1 tsp. celery seed
1 head cabbage sliced thin
Mix the vinegar, salad oil, sugar, salt,
dry mustard, celery seed and sugar.
Bring to a boil. Pour the boiled
mixture over the cabbage and stir.
Chill for 4 to 6 hours.
From the kitchen of Catherine G.

Sweet Sour Slaw

4- 6 slices bacon, crumbled

2 tbsp. onions, chopped

3 tbsp. bacon grease

¼ c. brown sugar

1 tsp. corn starch

¼ c. water

1 tsp. salt

¼ c. vinegar

4 c. cabbage, chopped

Sauté onions in bacon grease. Add sugar, cornstarch, salt, vinegar. Cool until thick. Combine in bowl with cabbage and crumbled bacon and dressing.

From the kitchen of Imodean D.

Cole Slaw

Head cabbage

Med. white or purple onion

Pint. sweet pickles

Pint. Hellman's Mayonnaise

1½ c. sugar

Salt to taste

Run first three ingredients through food processor. Add mayonnaise and sugar, mix well. Refrigerate 24 hours before serving. Keeps well in refrigerator for about one week.

From the kitchen of Melvin R.

"I believe that it isn't always enough to be forgiven by others. Sometimes you have to learn to forgive yourself."

Mother's Lime Cheese Salad

Lime cheese Salad.
1 pkg lime jello   2 - 3 oz pkge of cream cheese
1 c. hot water ½ c. pecans. 1 8. can of pineapple
1 c. or 8 large marshmellows
Dissolve jello, marshmellows & cream cheese in hot water add 1 c. of cold water, when thicken add pineapple & nuts.

From the kitchen of Irene T.

Taking the GAS-TRIC out of Beans

Bean-O works, but try taking the GAS-TRIC out of beans. Put a tablespoon of cooking oil in a pot of beans and one tablespoon of ginger. Cook until done. You can't taste the ginger. A sure thing. Pour over vegetables and refrigerate overnight. From the kitchen of Pat J.

Strawberry Spinach Salad Dressing

Dressing:

1 lemon

2 tbsp. white wine vinegar

1/3 c. sugar

1 tbsp. vegetable oil

1 tsp. poppy seeds

For dressing, zest lemon to measure ½ teaspoon zest. Juice lemon to measure 2 tablespoon juice. Combine zest, juice, vinegar, sugar, oil and poppy seeds. Whisk until well blended. Cover. Refrigerate until ready to use on spinach strawberry salad.

From the kitchen of Catherine G.

Spinach Salad

5 slices crisp bacon, crumbled

Big bag of spinach

¼ c. olive oil or canola oil

2 to 3 tbsp. of red wine vinegar

1 tbsp. lemon juice

½ tsp. sugar

¼ tsp. salt

Green onions

Mushrooms

Microwave bacon between paper towels 5-6 minutes to get dry crisp bacon. Let cool then crumble or with kitchen shears cut in small pieces and set aside. Wash and take stems off spinach. Add sliced green onions and mushrooms in the amount desired. Add bacon. Combine other ingredients in sauce pan and bring to boil. Pour over mixture and serve immediately. Add fresh ground pepper.

From the kitchen of Linda A.

It is impossible to live a positive life with a negative mind.

Korean Spinach Salad and Dressing

Dressing:

¾ c. sugar

1 c. salad oil

½ c. catsup

¼ c. vinegar

3 tbsp. Worcestershire Sauce

Medium onion, grated

Salt, dash

Mix the ingredients, making the dressing the day before.

Salad:

Pkg. fresh spinach (10 oz. or 1 lb.)

6 leaves of lettuce - torn

Can bean sprouts (drained)

5 bacon strips, fried and crumbled

2 eggs, hard boiled, chopped

Stir together in a salad bowl

Optional:

Add water chestnuts, sliced

From the kitchen of Catherine G.

Raw Cranberry Salad

2 c. ground cranberries

2 c. sugar

Apple, ground with skin

Orange, ground with rind

1 c. chopped nuts

1 c. boiling water

1 c. celery, diced

2 pkg. cherry jello (can substitute 1 pkg. lemon jello

Combine cranberries, apple, orange with sugar - let stand. Dissolve jello in water and add together with fruit immediately.   Add nuts and celery and chill until firm.

From the kitchen of Irene T.

Mandarin Salad

¼ c. sugar

Pkg. almonds

2 c. romaine

2 c. iceberg lettuce

1 c. chopped celery

Bunch green onions, finely chopped

Can mandarin oranges, drained and chilled

Sugared almonds

In a heavy skillet over med heat, mix sugar and almonds. Stir until sugar melts and barely starts to brown. Remove from skillet onto foil. After cooling, break apart. Mix next 5 ingredients and add sugared almonds

Sweet and Sour Dressing:

¼ c. oil

2 tbsp. sugar

2 tbsp. vinegar

1 tbsp. parsley

½ tsp. salt

dash of pepper

dash of red pepper sauce

Stir together and provide with salad

From the kitchen of Darlene B.

Salad Delight

3 c. shredded lettuce

1 c. grated raw cauliflower

½ c. grated carrots

3 tbsp. sweet relish

¼ tsp. vinegar

¼ tsp. olive oil

3 tbsp. sugar

½ tsp. salt

⅛ tsp. pepper

⅛ tsp. paprika

Combine lettuce, cauliflower, carrots and sweet relish in salad bowl. Stir together the other ingredients and pour over the salad and mix.

From the kitchen of Imodean D.

Taco Salad

Head lettuce, chopped

4 tomatoes, diced

Onion, chopped

Can chili beans

14 oz. grated cheese

1 lb. hamburger meat, fried and crumbled

Pkg. crushed Doritos

Place the chopped lettuce in a bowl. Stir in the tomatoes, onions, cheese and the meat. Stir in the Doritos

and place Doritos around the edge of the bowl.

From the kitchen of Imodean D.

Friend

Sometimes in life, you find a special friend;

Someone who changes your life just by being part of it.

Someone who makes you laugh until you can't stop;

Someone who makes you believe that there really is good in the world.

Someone who convinces you that there really is an unlocked door just waiting for you to open it.

This is Forever Friendship.

Author unknown

Mexican Chef Salad

Head of lettuce, cut up

Onion, chopped

4 tomatoes, chopped

8 oz. French dressing

Hot sauce

4 oz. grated cheddar cheese

Tortilla chips, large bag

Large avocado, sliced

1 lb. ground lean beef

Can (15 oz.) ranch style beans, drained

Toss lettuce, onion and tomatoes with cheese and French dressing and add hot sauce to taste. Crunch and add tortilla chips. Brown the beef, drain off any fat, and stir in beans. Simmer for 10 minutes, cool slightly, and mix into the cold salad. Decorate with more tortilla chips, avocado, and tomatoes. Serve immediately. Will not keep if left out. You may want to have French dressing and hot sauce separate and then have meat and beans in separate bowl.

From an unknown kitchen

Dash cayenne pepper
Line bottom of a micro-waveable plate with layers of paper towels. Stack bacon on paper towels in alternating layers. Microwave on HI until bacon is cooked. Layer bacon, cheese and onion in the bottom of dish. Beat together remaining ingredients and pour over cheese mixture. Microwave at MED-5 (50% power) for 20-25 minutes or just until center of quiche sets. Let stand for 5-8 minutes to complete cooking.

From the kitchen of Linda A.

Microwave Crustless Quiche Lorraine

½ lb. bacon, cooked and crumbled
Pkg. (4-oz) shredded cheddar cheese
¼ c. chopped green onions
4 eggs beaten
Can (13 oz) evaporated milk
¼ tsp. sugar, if desired
¼ tsp. salt

Woman's Perfect Breakfast

She's sitting at the table with her gourmet coffee.
Her son is on the cover of the Wheaties box.
Her daughter is on the cover of Business Week.
And her husband is on the back of the milk carton.

Special Chicken Salad

Red tipped leaf lettuce and Green leaf lettuce

1 to 2 - 13 oz. cans of chicken breasts, drained and flaked

Choose any two of the following fruits:

15 oz. can Mandarin oranges, drained

¾ c. sliced fresh strawberries

Red seedless grapes, amount desired

15 oz. can pineapples chucks or tidbits, drained

¼ to a c. sliced almonds and 1 c. or more of sliced celery

15 oz. chow mein noodles

Wash both lettuce. Spin out water. Tear lettuce into bit size pieces into a salad bowl. Add any two fruit choices, chicken breast, almonds, celery, and chow mein noodles. Toss salad and serve with a light vinaigrette or poppy seed dressing on the side. Do not add the chow mein noodles until time of serving.

From the kitchen of Linda A.

Mother's Sour Cream Salad

Sour Cream Salad

1 C sour cream   1 C chunked pineapple
1 C Mandrin oranges   1 C pecans
1 C cocoanut

Stir ingredients together & refrigate.

From the kitchen of Irene T.

Wilma's Cottage Cheese Jello Salad

Here's what's cookin'   Cottage Cheese Jello Salad.
Recipe from the kitchen of   Wilma VanGroningen.

2 pkgs orange Jello.
2½ c boiling water
½ c sugar
1 pinch of salt.
1 can (small) crushed pineapple

Let stand until cool & beat in carton of cottage cheese.
Fold in 1 cup of whipped cream or dream w hip.

From the kitchen of Wilma V.

"If you're headed in the wrong direction, God allows U-turns."

Cornbread Salad

Miracle Whip

Pan cornbread crumbled

Onion, chopped

2 - 4 green pepper, chopped

2 - 4 tomatoes, cut in small pieces

3 - 4 boiled eggs, chopped

4 - 6 slices bacon, crumbled

Mix together with Miracle Whip as desired.

Mother's Bread and Butter Pickles

Bread and Butter Pickles

Slice 25 to 30 Cucumbers

8 large onions

2 large Peppers   ½ C salt

Soak in Water 3 hrs - drain.

Pour in 5 C Vinegar

5 C sugar

2 T mustard seed

1 t turmeric

½ t cloves

Bring to boil - Pack in Jars.

From the kitchen of Irene T.

Pickled Beets

Cook beets until tender.

Fix a mixture of:

2 c. sugar

1 c. vinegar

Small amount of pickling spice

Drop beets into mixture and cook at medium heat (350° F.) a few minutes.   Add a little beet juice to mixture to make it red.

From the kitchen of Mildred A.

Sweet Dill Pickles

1 qt. dill pickle slices

2 - 2¾ c. sugar

1/3 c. vinegar

Combine the ingredients.

Leave at room temperature 4 hours. Stir occasionally. Pack in Pick-a-dill Tupperware and refrigerator.

Aunt Mabel's Beet Pickles

Beets to Pickle:

Select freshly gathered beets, about 1¼ inch diameter. If larger beets are used, quarter or slice after being cooked.   Cut off the tops of the beets, leaving 2 inch of stem. Leave the roots on. Wash thoroughly without breaking the skin so that the beets won't lose color.

Put in a kettle, cover with boiling water, and cook until the skin will slip off and the beets are done. (Do not overcook.)

Drain off the boiling water and

cover with cold water for a few minutes. Drain and peel the beets.

Spiced Vinegar:

Pint vinegar

½ c. water

½ c. sugar

1 tbsp. cinnamon

½ tbsp. allspice

6 cloves

Mix vinegar, water and sugar. Make a spice bag of cinnamon, allspice and cloves. Boil together. Pack beets into hot sterilized jars and cover with the hot spiced vinegar for pickle making. Use only good cider or fruit vinegar for making pickles. Poor vinegar ruins the color and good eating quality of pickles.

Packing Beets In Jars:

Fill jar with pickles, add hot spiced vinegar and place lid on good. Process quart jars 20 minutes at simmering temperatures in a hot water canner.

From the kitchen of Mabel K.

When you pray for others, God listens to you and blesses them; and sometimes, when you are safe and happy, remember that someone has prayed for you.

Wilma's Lime Pickles

7 lb. cucumbers sliced cross wise

1 c. lime

2 gal. water

4½ lb. sugar

2 pt. vinegar

1½ tbsp. salt

1 tsp. celery seed

1 tsp. whole cloves

2 tbsp. mixed pickling spice

Put cucumbers and lime in the water and let it stand for 24 hour, covered. Drain. Cover with fresh water for 3 hours covered Drain. Combine sugar, vinegar, salt, celery seed, cloves and pickling spice. Heat and pour over cucumbers and let stand all night or day - 12 hour. Drain liquid from pickles, heat drained liquid and boil for 35 minutes, Pour back over the cucumbers in jars. Seal and can. Make 6 or 7 pints. Best time to start is 4 or 5 p.m.

From the kitchen of Wilma V.

Lime Sweet Pickles

2 gal. water
2 c. lime
Add 7 lbs sliced cucumbers and soak 24 hrs.
Rinse well and drain, let set 3 to 4 hours.

Mix together:

9 c. sugar
2 qts. vinegar
1 tsp. pickling spice
2 tbsp. whole cloves
1 tsp. celery seeds
1 tsp. salt
Add to pickles and let stand overnight, then boil slow 35 minutes. Then pack and seal in jars.

Wilma's Chow-Chow

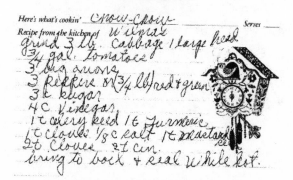

From the kitchen of Wilma V.

Stuffed Mushrooms

3 - 8 oz. cream cheese
1 c. Monterey Jack cheese
Garlic powder or minced garlic
Worcestershire sauce
12 slices of cooked bacon, crumbled large fresh mushrooms
Chop up stems of mushrooms and combine with other ingredients. Stuff mixture in mushrooms. Bake at 350° F for 15- 20 minutes.
From the kitchen of Phyllis T.

Minding My Own Business

I was walking past the mental hospital the other day.
All the patients were shouting, "13....13....13."
The fence was too high to see over, but I saw a little gap in the planks, so I looked through to see what was going on.
Somebody poked me in the eye with a stick!
Then they all started shouting "14...14....14"...

Meeting The Struggles Of Life

The Buzzard: If you put a buzzard in a pen that is 6 feet by 8 feet and is entirely open at the top, the bird, in spite of its ability to fly, will be an absolute prisoner. The reason is that a buzzard always begins a flight from the ground with a run of 10 to 12 feet. Without space to run, as is its habit, it will not even attempt to fly, but will remain a prisoner for life in a small jail with no top.

The Bat: The ordinary bat that flies around at night, a remarkably nimble creature in the air, cannot take off from a level place. If it is placed on the floor or flat ground, all it can do is shuffle about helplessly and, no doubt painfully, until it reaches some slight elevation from which it can throw itself into the air. Then, at once, it takes off like a flash.

The Bumble Bee: A bumble bee, if dropped into an open tumbler, will be there until it dies, unless it is taken out. It never sees the means of escape at the top, but persists in trying to find some way out through the sides near the bottom. It will seek a way where none exists, until it completely destroys itself.

People: In many ways, we are like the buzzard, the bat, and the bumble bee. We struggle about with all our problems and frustrations, never realizing that all we have to do is look up to God and seek his Holy Word.

Have a great day!

Author unknown

Chapter 8
Main Course Recipes

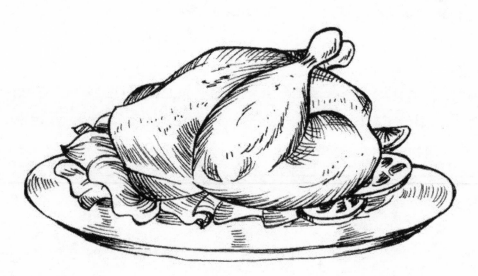

Index of Main Course Recipes

Chicken Pot Pie

Pillsbury Pie Crust placed in pie
    pan.
½ c. butter
Onion, sautéed
1 c. celery, chopped and sautéed
1 c. flour
¼ tsp. pepper
1 to 2 chicken bouillon cubes
Mix. **Add**:
1 c. water (I use the broth from
    my boiled chicken)
1 c. milk
3 c. diced chicken (cooked, boiled)
Cook and Stir until thick. Add: ½
small Package frozen uncooked
mix peas and carrots, 1 cup
partially boiled potatoes cut in
small cubes. Pour into pie crust
and cover with top crust. Bake at
425° F. for 25 to 30 minutes.
From the kitchen of Debbie W.

Happiness keeps You Sweet,
Trials keep You Strong,
Sorrows keep You Human,
Failures keep You Humble,
Success keeps You Glowing,
But Only God keeps You Going!
Author unknown

Easy Chicken Pot Pie

(As on Bisquick Box, but Modified)
2 c. frozen mixed vegetables,
    thawed
1 to 1½ c. cooked cut up chicken
    (may used canned)
Can cream of mushroom soup,
    low sodium
Can cream of chicken soup, low
    sodium
1 c. onions, chopped
Small can mushrooms, drained
    and rinsed

Heat oven to 400° F. Mix
chicken, soups, onions and
mushrooms. Pour into an ungreased 7-inch x 11-inch Pyrex or
large 9 inch deep dish pie plate.
Stir together until moistened:
1 c. Bisquick
½ c. milk
1 egg, beaten
Dolop on top of chicken mixture.
Bake 30 minutes until golden
brown. Serves approximately six.
Modified from a box of Bisquick.
From the kitchen of Linda A.

Chicken Tetrazzini

2-3 bacon strips
½ c. chopped bell pepper
½ c. chopped onion
Small can of sliced mushrooms-
    drained
Small jar of pimentos
2 tbsp. flour
Can chicken broth
Can (16 oz.) evaporated milk
2 c. diced, cooked chicken
12 oz. cooked spaghetti noodles
Parmesan cheese
Fry bacon in skillet, remove bacon and crumble into bits. Cook bell pepper and onion in bacon grease until tender. Add mushrooms, pimentos, flour, and chicken broth. Cook mixture until it begins to thicken. Add bacon bits, can of milk, and chicken. Pour mixture over noodles in a baking dish. Bake at 350° F. for 30 minutes. or until hot and bubbly. Sprinkle with cheese and serve.
From the kitchen of. Alecia M.

May peace break into your home and may thieves come to steal your debts.

Chicken Tetrazzini

6 lb. hen, chopped
1 c. mushrooms, chopped
1 c. onions, chopped
1 c. peppers, chopped
1 c. celery, chopped
2 cans mushroom soup
Small can pimento
Small can ripe olives
Can cream of chicken soup
2 cans of chicken broth
1 c. cheddar cheese, grated
½ lb spaghetti (½ of 1 box)
Sauté onions, peppers, celery in butter. Add mushroom soup and 2 cans of chicken broth. Add chopped chicken cut into bit size pieces. Add chopped mushrooms. Add chicken soup. Add this to spaghetti that has been cooked in chicken broth. Add pimento, olives, cheddar cheese. Mix well. In oven, heat until cheese is melted. If too thick, add more broth.
From the kitchen of Thel H.

Barbecued Chicken

½ c. flour
½ tsp. salt, if desired
1 tsp. paprika
¼ tsp. pepper
8 chicken breast, sliced diagonally
    or 16 chicken tenders

Preheat oven to 350° F. Mix flour, salt, paprika, and pepper. Coat chicken pieces with flour mixture. Fry the chicken in a frying pan until brown. Place the chicken in a 13-inch x 9-inch x 2-inch baking dish. Spoon hot barbecue sauce over the chicken. Cover the dish with tin foil. Bake for 45 minutes.

Barbecue Sauce:

1 c. catsup or 8 oz. of tomato
    sauce
½ c. hot water
2 tsp. paprika
1/3 c. lemon juice
½ tsp. salt, if desired
2 tbsp. Worcestershire sauce
1 medium onion, finely chopped

Mix all ingredients and heat to boiling, stirring the sauce occasionally.

From the kitchen of Aukse H.

Oven Baked Chicken

Half one whole chicken
Sprinkle front and back with salt, garlic powder and soy sauce.
Bake at 400° F, turning once, for one hour to two hour and 30 minutes, depending on the size of the chicken. Better than Boston Market.

From the kitchen of Paula H.

Oven Baked Chicken

Pkg. of Hidden Valley Ranch
    Dressing
1 c. parmesan cheese
1 c. crushed cornflakes
½ c. melted butter or margarine
1 lb. chicken tenders or breast

Mix the Ranch Dressing mix, cheese and cornflakes together in a plastic bag. Melt butter in a shallow bowl. Dip the chicken in the butter then toss in the bag.
Bake at 350° F. for 30 minutes or until juices run clear.

Monterey Chicken-Rice Bake

2 c. cottage cheese
2 c. sour cream
1 tsp. garlic powder
¾ c. coarsely crushed corn chips (Fritos)
1 tsp. salt
3 oz. of softened cream cheese
1 c. shredded Monterey Jack cheese
Can cream of chicken soup
Can (16 oz.) chopped tomatoes
8 oz. of diced green chilies
3 c. cooked chicken, diced
3 c. cooked rice

Blend together cottage cheese, cream cheese, and sour cream until smooth. Add rest of ingredients-except crushed chips. Pour mixture into a baking dish and sprinkle with the chips. Bake 20-30 minutes at 350° F.
From the kitchen of Alecia M.

Teriyaki Chicken and Vegetables

8 Individually frozen, boneless, skinless chicken tenderloins
3 tbsp. vegetable oil
1 pkg. (8 oz.) raw broccoli florets
½ cup water
½ c. sliced carrots
½ c. chopped celery and 1 sm.
Pkg. fresh mushrooms
½ c. zucchini squash and ½ c. yellow squash
Bottle thick teriyaki sauce

Rinse frozen chicken tenderloins with cold water and pat dry. Heat oil in a large nonstick skillet. Stir fry vegetables until tender crisp and transfer to bowl. Add chicken and water to skillet. Cover, cook over med. heat until done. Return vegetables to the skillet, add teriyaki sauce. Stir fry over high heat until heated through. Serve over white rice.
From the kitchen of Debbie W.

Don't go for looks; they can deceive. Don't go for wealth; even that fades away. Go for someone who makes you smile, because it takes only a smile to make a dark day seem bright. Find the one that makes your heart smile.

Chicken Ritz

Chicken or three chicken breasts
Can of cream of chicken
Can of cream of celery
Small container of sour cream
1 tube of Ritz crackers
½ c. butter, melted
Boil chicken or chicken breasts. Remove bones and chop into small chunks. Mix the chunks with the chicken soup, celery soup (Do not add water) and the sour cream. Stir this together and pour into a casserole dish that has been sprayed with Pam. Smash the Ritz crackers in the tube by hand until they are crumbs. Open the tube and spread over chicken mixture. Drizzle the melted butter over the crackers in casserole. Cook uncovered in oven at 350° F. for 20 - 30 minutes until it is bubbling. (You can use non fat sour cream and also the butter is optional, making it less fattening.)
From the kitchen of Mildred A.

Sauerkraut and Chicken

1 lb. sauerkraut
2 tbsp. brown sugar
1 sliced apple or ½ c. applesauce
3 chicken leg quarters [remove skin and all visible fat]
Black pepper
Put sauerkraut in bottom of crock pot, top with apple and brown sugar. Lay chicken on top, sprinkle with pepper. Slow cook on medium heat 6 – 8 hours. (Can also be cooked on top of stove in Dutch oven for 2 hours). Makes 4 servings.
From the kitchen of June T.

Chicken Loaf

2 lb. chicken diced (pre-cooked)
1 c. fresh bread crumbs
½ c. rice (measure after cooked)
¼ tsp. salt
1 tbsp. pimento, chopped
1½ c. milk or chicken broth
2 eggs, beaten
Mix ingredients, adding eggs last. Bake 1 hour in a low heat oven at 300° F.
From the kitchen of Imodean D.

Poppy Seed Chicken

8 boneless chicken breast (Cooked and diced)
2 can cream mushroom soup and 8 oz. sour cream
2 c. crushed Ritz crackers (42-44 crackers)
3 tbsp. poppy seeds
Stick butter, melted

Heat and pour the soup over the chicken in a 9-inch x 13-inch pan. Stir in the sour cream. Mix the crackers and poppy seeds and spread over the chicken mixture. Drizzle the butter over the crackers. Bake for 20 minutes at 350° F.

From the kitchen of Claudia W.

Clay Pot Chicken Leeks Sommers

4 large leeks, washed, halved, green, top removed
Chicken: 3 lbs. cut up, skin removed or chicken breasts
3 tbsp. cumin
salt and black pepper
3 tbsp. butter
3 c. chicken broth
½ tsp. garlic or more
Dutch oven or soaked clay pot in

325° F. oven. Line bottom of pot with leeks, then chicken, and put in ½ of cumin, salt, pepper, and butter. Layer again with leeks, chicken, spices, dot with butter and put additional layer of leeks over top. Pour broth over it. Cover and bake two hours. Yummy. May put baked garlic over chicken.

From the kitchen of Paula H.

June's Chicken Enchiladas

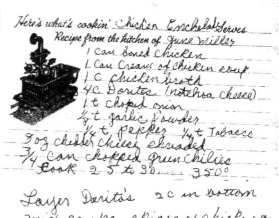

Here's what's cookin' Chicken Enchelat Serves
Recipe from the kitchen of June Miller
1 can boned chicken
1 Can Cream of chicken soup
1 c chicken broth
4 c Doritos (notchos cheese)
1 t choped onion
½ t garlic powder
¼ t pepper   ¼ t Tabasco
3 oz chedder cheese shreaded
¾ can chopped green chilies
Cook 25 to 30   350°

Layer Doritos   2 c in bottom
mix soups, spices & chicken & Chillies
Pour half over doritos repeat.
cover with cheese.

From the kitchen of Irene T.

Microwave Chicken or Turkey Enchiladas

6 corn tortillas (If frozen, defrost by placing between paper towels and microwave on HI for 45 to 60 seconds.)

Filling:

2 c. chicken or turkey, cooked & cubed

½ tsp. salt

8 oz. ricotta or cottage cheese

⅛ tsp. pepper

½ c. ripe olives, chopped

⅛ tsp. garlic powder

2 tsp. parsley flakes

Sauce:

Medium onion, chopped

2 tsp. chili powder

½ med. green pepper, chopped

1 tsp. sugar

15 oz. can tomato sauce

⅛ tsp. garlic powder

7 oz. green chilies, drained & chopped, optional

Topping:

1½ c. shredded Cheddar cheese

Combine filling ingredients in medium mixing bowl. Divide evenly into 6 portions. Place one portion of filling down center of each tortilla. Roll up. Arrange seam side down in 12-inch x 9-inch dish. Combine onion and green pepper in 1½ quart casserole. Cover. Microwave on HI three to four minutes, or till vegetables are tender. Stir in remaining sauce ingredients. Pour over filled tortillas. Cover with wax paper. Microwave on HI for 7 - 10 minutes, or until heated through. Sprinkle with cheddar cheese. Reduce power to 50% (MED). Microwave uncovered three to five minutes, or until cheese melts. Serves 4-6. From the kitchen of Linda A.

Share

You were taught to share when you were only two years old. When did you forget? That rule still applies. Share with those who are less fortunate than you. Share your joy with those who need encouragement. Share your laughter with those who haven't heard any in such a long time. Share your tears with those who have forgotten how to cry. Share your faith with those who have none. Author Unknown.

Chicken Enchiladas

Pkg. (8 oz.) Philadelphia cream cheese

19-20 oz. canned chicken breast

½ c. green pepper

½ c red pepper

½ small can (2 oz.) chopped green chilies

¾. lb Velveeta pasteurized cheese spread

8 oz. Salsa

8 large whole wheat tortillas

Stir chicken, peppers and cream cheese and about 3 ounces of Salsa in saucepan on low heat until cream cheese is melted. Spoon chicken mixture down the center of each tortilla and roll them up and place them in a 9-inch x 13-inch baking dish. Stir Velveeta and milk in sauce pan, on low until smooth. Then pour over rolled tortillas and bake for 20 minutes at 350° F. Cover with rest of salsa.

From the kitchen of Paula H.

King Ranch Casserole

Can Rotel tomatoes

Can mushroom soup

Can cream of chicken soup or (¼

1 c. butter

¼ c. flour

1½ c. chicken broth)

Chicken

Can chicken broth

Onion

½ green pepper

1 lb. American cheese (or 12 oz. Velveeta)

Dozen Tortillas

Make a sauce of tomatoes, mushroom soup, cream of chicken and broth. Boil, de-bone and cut up the chicken into bite size pieces. In a 9-inch x 13-inch casserole dish, make a layer of tortilla, chicken, onions, green pepper, cheese. Repeat. Pour sauce over all and bake at 350° F. for 15 minutes or more.

From the kitchen of Paula H.

Everything Jambalaya

2 c. enriched white rice

1 tbsp. extra virgin olive oil

1 tbsp. butter

1 lb. boneless, skinless chicken, cubed

¾ lb. andouille sausage, casing removed and diced

Medium onion, chopped

2 ribs celery, chopped

Green bell pepper, chopped

Bay leaf, fresh or dried

2 tbsp. cayenne pepper sauce

2-3 tbsp. flour

Can (14 oz.) diced tomatoes in juice

Can (14 oz.) of chicken broth

1 tsp. cumin

1 tsp. rounded dark chili powder

1 tsp. poultry seasoning

1 tsp. Worcestershire sauce

1 lb. med shrimp, raw, de-veined and peeled

scallion and thyme chopped for garnish

Cook rice according to package. directions. Place a large, deep skillet over med. high heat. Add oil and butter to the pan. Cube chicken and place in hot oil and butter. Brown chicken three minutes. Add sausage, and cook two minutes more. Add onion, celery, pepper, bay leaf, and cayenne. Sauté vegetables for five minutes, sprinkle flour over the pan and cook 1-2 minutes more. Stir in tomatoes and broth and season with cumin, chili, poultry seasoning, and Worcestershire. Bring liquids to a boil and add shrimp. Simmer shrimp five minutes until pink and firm. From the kitchen of Alecia M.

Hawaiian Beef

3 to 4 lb. cross cut beef shanks (use shoulder roast, arm roast, or stew meat)

3 tbsp. vegetable oil

½ c. water

¼ c. light soy sauce

Medium onion, sliced

¼ tsp. pepper and ¼ tsp. ginger

4 oz. can mushroom stems and pieces (optional)

Can (9 oz. or more) pineapple chunks and natural juice

1/3 c. sliced celery

Fresh green beans (enough for ½ c. + per guest)

¼ c. water

2 tbsp. flour
Brown meat slightly in oil. Add soy sauce, ½ c. water, pepper, ginger, and onion. Cover tightly and cook very slowly 2½ to 3 hours or until meat is tender. Add a little more water if necessary. Add mushrooms, pineapple, celery, and green beans. Continue cooking 20 to 30 minutes or until celery and green beans are tender. Remove meat to a heated platter and green beans to a covered bowl. Mix ¼ c. water and flour. Add to cooking liquid and cook, stirring constantly until thickened. Serve gravy with meat. Cook 1½ cup of rice and serve the Hawaiian Beef over the rice. Serve with salad and hot bread.
Serves 8 to 10.
From the kitchen of Linda A.

God doesn't call the qualified, He qualifies the called.

Paula's Chicken Fried Steak

4 cubed, tenderized beef steaks.
Salt and pepper.
Dip twice into mixture of two beaten eggs and milk, then flour. Fry in canola oil. Serve with brown gravy from the pan drippings.
From the kitchen of Paula H.

Mother's Pot Roast

Arm Roast
Salt and pepper
Brown on both sides in 2 tablespoon oil. Cover with water. Add one-quartered onion. Cover and simmer for 4 hours. Add carrots and potatoes last 30 minutes. Make gravy from water and flour added to pan juices.
From the kitchen of Irene T.

Stromboli

Loaf frozen bread dough
Ounce of sliced pepperoni (I use
  turkey pepperoni)
¾ lb. browned sausage
4 oz. shredded Mozzarella cheese
4 oz. shredded Cheddar cheese
Onions
Green peppers
Mushrooms
Olives (Optional
Parmesan Cheese
Spaghetti sauce
Thaw bread dough and let rise to
double size. Spread out dough on
a lightly greased cookie sheet.
Layer down the center the
sausage, pepperoni, onions, green
peppers, mushrooms that have
been sautéed slightly, and cheeses.
Fold ends together, pinching
tightly to enclose it all.   Flip over
so seam is on the bottom.   Baste
the top with butter and sprinkle
with Parmesan cheese.   Bake at
350° F. for about 25 minutes.
Slice and serve with warm
spaghetti sauce and Parmesan
cheese.
From the kitchen of Ruth B.

Brisket

1 tbsp. liquid smoke
2 tbsp. Worcestershire sauce
2 tbsp. soy sauce
1 tsp. garlic salt
1 tsp. onion salt
2 tsp. celery salt
1 tsp. salt
1 tsp. pepper
Put brisket in foil envelope. Mix
above ingredients together and
pour over meat and seal envelope.
It can be marinated in the
refrigerator overnight or cooked
immediately. Bake at 275° F. for
4-6 hours, depending upon the
size of your brisket. This is also
great served as BBQ sandwiches.
Prepare as stated above then chop
up meat and pour your favorite
BBQ sauce over; serve on
hamburger buns.
From the kitchen of Catherine G.

Brisket Marinade

(Modified)

Combine:
1 tbsp. liquid smoke
2 tbsp. light soy sauce
2 tbsp. Worshershire sauce
1 tsp. garlic powder
1 tsp. onion powder
1 tsp. pepper
2 tsp. celery salt
Use meat fork and make many stabs in a 4 lb. fresh brisket - on both sides. Remove excess fat. Place brisket in foil inside baking dish. Pour marinade over the brisket. Wrap and refrigerate overnight. May flip foil over once or twice. Leave in aluminum foil in the baking dish and bake for five hours at 275° F.
From the kitchen of Catherine G. and modified by Linda A.

Michael's Cholent

1 whole green jalapeno chopped up or whole just for flavor
1 lb. cubed meat
1 c. dried beans - pick your favorite
½ clove garlic
3 large potatoes
1 c. barley
½ bag baby carrots
Whole onion - chopped up in small pieces
Stir the ingredients and add water to bring crock pot to ¾ full.
Cook on high for 2 hr then on low overnight.
NOTES:
Also if desired:
add more meat.
add ½ c. of barbeque sauce for extra flavor.
extra potatoes.
Add favorite spices.
Add ¼ c. oil to bottom of crock pot before filling.
From the Kitchen of Michael A.

Love Yourself

As much as I love you, how can you not love yourself? You were created by me for one reason only -- to be loved, and to love in return. I am a God of Love. Love Me. Love your neighbors. But also love yourself. It makes My heart ache when I see you so angry with yourself when things go wrong. You are very precious

to me.   Don't ever forget......
Touch someone with your love.
Rather than focus upon the thorns
of life, smell the roses and count
your blessings
Author unknown

Teriyaki

2 lbs. flank steak, sliced thin
½ c. chopped onion
Cloves garlic, crushed
4 tbsp. soy sauce
2 tbsp. salad oil
2 tbsp. brown sugar
½ tbsp. black pepper
2 tbsp. dry sherry (optional)
2 cans (8½ oz. each) water
   chestnuts
Trim steak, slice on angle across
grain in very thin slices. Mix all
ingredients except steak and water
chestnuts.   Wrap each chestnut in
slice of steak, using toothpicks.
Marinate in refrigerator for 2
hours. Broil 4 inches from heat
for 2-3 minutes.
From the kitchen of Janet K.

Microwave Layered Florentine Wild Rice With Beef and Olives

1½ lbs. ground, lean beef
Onion, chopped
4 oz. can sliced mushrooms
4 oz. can black olives
1 tsp. Italian dressing
¼ tsp. garlic powder
1 tsp. fajita season
2 - 10 oz. pkg. frozen chopped
   spinach, thawed and drained
3-4 Roma tomatoes, sliced or
   chopped
Pkg. Mabatma Wild Rice Mix
Pkg. Success Rice
Pkg. Pioneer Gravy Mix, No Fat
Country or No Fat Chicken
   prepared according to
   directions on the pkg. (2 cups)
8 oz. grated Kraft 4 cheese mix
4 oz. parmesan cheese
Crumble beef into plastic colander
set over a glass catch bowl.
Microwave on HI for 5 minutes,
stir, cook 5 more minutes on HI.
Sauté onion and mushrooms, in
small amount of oil. Add olives
and seasoning.   Combine with
meat mixture in large bowl and
toss. Prepare Mahatma and

Success rice according to package directions, combine in bowl, set aside. Prepare gravy mix according to directions, set aside. Line 9 inch x 13 inch casserole with Baker's Mate. Layer half of the rice, all of the spinach, remaining rice,

1 c. of shredded 4 cheese mixture, cover with

1 c. of prepared gravy mix. Add layer of meat mixture, then tomatoes and remaining 1 c. of gravy. Cook 8 minutes on HI and 12 minutes on MED in microwave or 40 minutes in a 350° F. oven. Top with remaining 1 cup cheese and sprinkle with parmesan cheese.

From the kitchen of Linda A.

Stuffed Cabbage Rolls

2 lb. ground meat, lean
1 c. rice
2 - 6 oz. cans tomato paste
1 clove garlic
½ stick oleo
1½ tsp. salt
2 tsp. black pepper
1 tsp. cayenne
3 tsp. cummin
1 large cabbage head
Blend ingredients with hands.
Place cabbage in pot of boiling

water for only a few seconds. Peel one leaf at a time. Split leaves in halves down the vein. Roll mixture in the leaves. Seal with toothpicks, if you like. Put leaves in bottom of pan, packing tightly. Cover with cabbage leaves. Cover with water and bring to boil. Simmer for 25 minutes.

From the kitchen of Paula H.

Be Patient

I managed to fix it so in just one lifetime you could have so many diverse experiences. You grow from a child to an adult, have children, change jobs many times, learn many trades, travel to so many places, meet thousands of people, and experience so much. How can you be so impatient then when it takes Me a little longer than you expect to handle something on My to-do-list? Trust in My timing, for My timing is perfect. Just because I created the entire universe in only six days, everyone thinks I should always rush, rush, rush.

Author Unknown

Lasagna

1 lb. ground meat

1 clove garlic, minced

1 tbsp. whole basil and ½ tsp. salt

1 lb. can tomatoes

2 - 6 oz. cans tomato paste

10 oz. Lasagna noodles (You may not use all the box.)

3 c. Ricotta cheese

½ c. grated Romano or Parmesan cheese

2 eggs, beaten and ½ tsp. pepper

2 tbsp. parsley flakes

1 lb. Mozzarella cheese, sliced thin

Heat oven to 375° F. Brown meat slowly. Spoon off fat. Add the next five ingredients. Simmer, uncovered, 30 minutes. Stir occasionally. Cook noodles as directed on the package. Drain and rinse. Combine the remaining ingredients, except the Mozzarella cheese. Place half the noodles in oblong baking dish. Spread with half the Ricotta cheese mixture. Add half of the Mozzarella and then the meat sauce. Repeat layers. Bake at 375° F. for 30 minutes. Let stand ten minutes before cutting into squares.

From the kitchen of Paula H.

Debbie's Lasagna

1 to 1½ lb. extra lean ground beef

2 – 8 oz. cans tomato sauce

2 – 8 oz. can water or (green tea)

6 oz. can tomato paste

24 oz. sm. Curd cottage cheese

32 oz. pkg. shredded Mozzarella cheese

20 oz. box Oven Ready Lasagna Noodles:

Brown ground beef, add a little salt, pepper, garlic powder and a small chopped onion. Drain any fat. Blend together tomato sauce, tomato paste and 2 cans of water. Add the following spices to your taste:

1 tsp. garlic

Salt and pepper if more is needed

1 tbsp. basil

2 bay leaves

½ tsp. oregano - Mrs. Dash (Original blend)

Let simmer at very low heat for about 20 minutes. Blend cottage cheese. Layer in 13 inch x 9 inch pan begin with a little meat mixture and remove bay leaves, when you come across them. Add some cottage cheese then sprinkle mozzarella then place uncooked noodles, continue to alternate and make sure you end with meat mixture and top with remaining mozzarella then sprinkle parmesan cheese and parsley flakes on the top. Bake at 375° F. for about 45 minutes to one hour.

From the kitchen of Debbie W.

Bierocks

Dough:

2 tbsp. active dry yeast
½ c. lukewarm water
1½ c. lukewarm milk
½ c. shortening
½ c. sugar
2 eggs
1 tsp. salt
3½ c. flour

Stir together and roll out the dough and divide into 7 inches diagonal round . (This could be used with fried pies as well) [and the lazy cook's alternative is to purchase frozen bread dinner rolls and roll them out for the same use.]

Filling:

1 lb. lean ground beef, browned
Med. head cabbage, chopped
Large onion, chopped
2 cloves of garlic
Salt to taste

Cook these ingredients together.

Let them cool and then place them on the cutout dough or dinner rolls. With the filling on the dough, fold it over and pinch together the edge. Set each one, with the pinched side up, in baking dishes and bake for 15 - 20 minutes at 350° F.

From the kitchen of Mildred A.

Beef Porcupines

Pkg. beef Rice a Rona
1 lb. ground beef
1 egg, beaten
Beef seasoning, from Rice-a-Rona
    package.
2½ c. hot water
Flour

Combine Rice a Rona, beef and egg and shape into balls. Brown in small amount of oil and drain if any is left. Combine beef seasoning with hot water and pour over meat . Cover and simmer for 30 minutes. Thicken with a water and flour mixture. Serve with mashed potatoes.

From the kitchen of Paula H.

Microwave Texas Meatballs and Rice

1 lb. ground beef
1 egg, slightly beaten
1½ tsp. chili powder
1 tsp. salt and ¼ tsp. pepper
Can (16 oz.) stewed tomatoes
1 large onion, thinly sliced and
    separated into rings
Large green pepper, chopped
¾ c. uncooked instant rice
Mix ground beef, egg, chili powder, salt and pepper. Shape into 1½ to 2 inch balls. Place in 2 quart casserole. Microwave at HI (100%) until meatballs are set and lose pink color, 4 - 7 minutes, rearranging meatballs after half the cooking time, Drain. Stir in the remaining ingredients; cover. Microwave at HI (100%) until mixture is bubbly and onions are tender, 4 - 7 minutes. Stir after half the cooking time. Let stand until rice is tender, 2 - 3 minutes. Makes 4 servings.
From the kitchen of Linda A.

Hamburger Stroganoff

½ c. minced onion
1 clove garlic, minced
¼ c. butter or olive oil

1 lb. ground beef, very lean
2 tbsp. flour
¼ tsp. pepper
Can (8 oz.) sliced mushrooms,
    drained
Can cream of chicken soup,
    undiluted
1 c. commercial sour cream
Sauté onion and garlic in butter over medium stove top heat, remove from pan. Brown meat and drain fat, add onion and garlic back to the pan. Stir in flour, pepper, and mushrooms. Cook 5 minutes. Add small amount of water if needed. Stir in soup. Simmer uncovered for 10 minutes. Stir in sour cream. Heat thoroughly. Serve with rice or noodles.
From the kitchen of Linda A.

Microwave Hamburger Pie

Crust:
1 lb. lean ground beef
1 tbsp. dry mustard
1 egg
¼ tsp. ground cumin
¼ c. dry bread crumbs
1 tsp. garlic powder
1 tbsp. light soy sauce

Filling:
1½ c. sliced potatoes
¾ c. sliced onion, (1/8 in. thick)
    separated into rings.
1 c. sliced mushrooms
Topping:
1 c. shredded Cheddar cheese
½ c. shredded Swiss cheese
1½ tsp. parsley flakes
Combine all crust ingredients and mix well.   Press into a deep 9-inch pie pan.   Microwave at HI three to five minutes or until meat is set (some pink may remain), rotating once or twice during cooking. Drain. Top meat with a layer of potato slices; follow with onions, and then with mushrooms. Cover with wax paper. Microwave at HI 4½ to 8½ minutes or until potatoes in center are fork tender, rotating once during cooking. Reduce power to 50% (MED). Sprinkle with cheese and parsley. Microwave, uncovered, two to five minutes (MED) or until cheese melts. Let stand two to three minutes before serving. Serves 4-6.
From the kitchen of Linda A.

Beans and Hamburger Casserole Large

5 cans pinto beans
5 cans ranch style beans
4 lb. hamburger meat
3 medium onions, chopped
1 c. catsup
½ c. mustard
½ c. dark syrup
1 c. brown sugar
Brown the meat and onions together, then stir in the other ingredients. Cover and cook at 250° F. for about 1 hour.
From the Kitchen of Melba R.

Beans and Hamburger Casserole Small

Can pinto beans
Can ranch style beans
1 lb. hamburger
¾ c. onion, chopped
¼ c. catsup
2 tbsp. mustard
2 tbsp. dark syrup
¼ c. brown sugar
Brown the meat and onions. Stir in the other ingredients. Cover and cook at 250° F. for about 1 hour.
From the kitchen of Melba R.

Hamburger Casserole

1¼ lb. beef (browned & drained)
Can cream mushroom soup and 1
Can Durkee French fried onions
Grated cheddar cheese (as much
    as you like)
Bag tater tots
Stir the soup into the cooked beef.
Layer the other ingredients in
order in a greased 9-inch x 13-inch
pan. Bake at 350° F. for 50
minutes.

Hamburger Casserole

1 lb. ground meat
2 eggs, beaten
Carrot, grated
Large potato, grated
Some garlic salt or powder
Pkg. saltine crackers
Mix together and make into
meatballs and brown. Put into a
casserole dish. Mix one can of
mushroom soup with one can of
milk. Pour over the meat balls
and bake for 30 minutes at 350° F.
From the kitchen of Pat J.

Tallerina

1 med. pepper, chopped
1 lb. hamburger
1 tbsp. oil and 1 tsp. chili powder
Stir together and brown.
Salt and pepper to taste
ADD AND STIR IN:
1 cooked pkg. egg noodles (50)
1 lb. Velveeta, grated
Can tomatoes
Can whole kernel corn
Jar olives and brine (22 olives,
    less than ¼ c. brine) Serve
    with crackers.
From the kitchen of Corrine T.

Baked Chili

1 lb. + hamburger, lean
1 c. celery, chopped
¾ c. onion, chopped
½ c. green pepper, chopped
½ c. egg plant or summer squash
2 tbsp. oil
2 cloves garlic
2 tsp. chili
½ tsp. cumin
½ tsp. pepper
½ tsp. crushed red pepper seeds
15 oz. can tomato sauce
15 oz. can stewed or crushed
    tomatoes
1 or 2 cans chili beans with liquid
1 can butter beans or cannellini
beans, rinsed and drained. Brown
and drain the hamburger and put
in a side dish. In the skillet, cook

the celery, onion, green pepper, egg plant/squash and garlic in the oil. Add the hamburger back into the skillet or pot. Add the chili, cumin, pepper, crushed pepper and tomato products and cook for about 10 minutes. Add cans of chili beans and butter bean, heat oven to 350° F. <u>Prepare Jiffy Cornbread as box instructs.</u> Oil 2 - 2½ quart casseroles and heat in oven. Pour the jiffy mix into the 2 heated casserole bowls. Pour chili mixture on top of the cornbread and bake for 20 minutes. Add one cup or more grated cheese to top and bake 10 minutes longer. Makes 8-12 servings

From the kitchen of Aukse H.

Chili

5 lbs. chili meat, such as, hamburger
2 or more cloves of garlic, chopped fine
¼ c. or more canola oil
2 pkg. of Uncle William's Chili Mix
3 tbsp. chili powder
3 cans tomato sauce
2 cans water

Brown meat in canola oil. Add garlic and cook until meat is not pink. Add chili mix, chili powder. Cook about 10 minutes. Add tomato sauce and water. Cook until meat is tender. You may have to add a little more water as it cooks down.

From the kitchen of Mildred A.

Green Chili Enchiladas

Dozen corn tortillas
½ c. cooking oil
2 c. Monterey Jack cheese, shredded
¾ c. chopped onion
¼ c. butter or margarine
¼ c. flour
2 c. chicken broth
1 c. sour cream
5-7 jalapeno peppers, seeded and chopped

In skillet, cook tortillas in hot oil for 15 seconds on each side. Put 2 tablespoon. cheese and 1 tbsp. onion on each tortilla. Place seam down, in oblong baking dish. In sauce pan, melt butter or margarine. Blend in flour. Add chicken broth. Cook, stirring constantly, until thick and bubbly. Then remove from the heat. Stir in sour cream and jalapenos. Pour over tortillas. Bake as 425° F. for 20 minutes. Sprinkle remaining cheese on top and bake for 5 minutes more.

From the kitchen of Paula H.

Green Chili Enchiladas

Sauce (4 c.):
¼ c. vegetable or olive oil
Onion, chopped
2-3 garlic cloves, chopped
¼ c. four
½ tsp. ground cumin
½ tsp. black pepper
3 c. chicken broth
1 c. green chili, chopped
½ tsp. oregano
1 tsp. salt
Shredded Monterrey Jack Cheese
Heat oil in 3 quart saucepan over medium heat. Add onion and garlic, cover and cook over low heat about 5 minutes to wilt onions. Raise heat to medium again, stir in flour, cumin and black pepper and cook, stirring for 2 minutes (or more) to cook rawness out of flour. It may clump, but that's okay. When it begins to color, remove from heat and whisk in broth. Add all remaining ingredients. Return pan to heat and bring to boiling point, then cover and simmer over low heat for 30 minutes, stirring occasionally. The finished sauce should be thick enough to nap on a spoon - can dilute with water.

Enchiladas:
Dip each corn tortilla in hot oil and brown, then add sauce, and add shredded Monterrey Jack Cheese and roll up. A 9 inch x 13 inch pan will hold 12 tortillas. Cover ends (and more) with sauce and put remainder of cheese in middle of enchiladas. Bake 15 minutes at 350° F.

From the kitchen of Catherine G.

Chili Rellenos Casserole

1 lb. grated cheddar
½ lb. Monterey jack
1 lg. can (27 oz.) Ortega Whole Green Chili
4 eggs
4 tbsp. flour
1 tsp. salt
Large can of evaporated milk
Remove stems and seeds from chili peppers. Line greased 9-inch x 13-inch dish with one layer of peppers. Cover with half of

mixed grated cheese. Add another layer of peppers and the remaining cheese. Beat the eggs, mix in the flour, salt and evaporated milk. Beat until smooth. Pour evenly over peppers and cheese. Bake 45 minutes at 350° F. until custard is set and a golden brown. Serve with Picante sauce.

From the kitchen of Catherine G.

Panhandle Casserole

1 lb. lean sausage

Can green chopped chilies, undrained

1¼ lb. Monterrey Jack cheese, or a blend of cheese, grated

9 eggs, beaten

1 c. milk or Milnot

2 tbsp. flour

Brown sausage and drain between paper towels. Layer sausage with cheeses and chopped chilies in a 9-inch x 13-inch glass baking dish. Combine eggs, milk and flour until well blended. Pour liquid over layered mixtures. Cook at 350° F. for 30 to 45 minutes. Slice and serve.

From the kitchen of Elizabeth B.

Sopa De Fideo

3 tbsp. oil

8 oz. spaghetti, thin

1 lb. lean hamburger meat

2 c. celery, sliced

2 c. onion, sliced

½ c. green pepper, chopped

16 oz. can of corn

1 c. water

1 tbsp. or more chili powder

½ tsp. or more garlic powder

32 oz. can tomatoes, blended or cut up

Add salt if desired

1/8 tsp. cayenne pepper

8 oz. sliced or shredded cheese

In an electric skillet, brown uncooked spaghetti (break in half) in oil (at 275° F.) Remove from the skillet. Brown hamburger in skillet. Remove any excess grease. Add spaghetti and remaining ingredients (except cheese). Bring to a simmer and cook covered, for 25 minutes. Add more water if needed. Add cheese. Cover and simmer till cheese melts. Add parsley and serve. Serves 8.

From the Kitchen of Linda A.

Spaghetti Pie

6 oz. spaghetti
2 tbsp. butter
½ c. grated Parmesan cheese
2 eggs, beaten
1 lb. ground beef or pork
    sausage
½ c. chopped onion
¼ c. green bell pepper, chopped
18 oz. can tomatoes cut up
16 oz. can tomato paste
1 tsp. sugar
1 tsp. dried oregano
¼ tsp. garlic salt
1 c. cottage cheese
½ c. Mozzarella cheese shredded

Cook spaghetti according to package directions; drain. Stir butter into hot spaghetti. Add parmesan cheese and eggs. Put spaghetti mixture into buttered 10 inch pie plate to form crust. In skillet brown meat with onion, green peppers until vegetables are tender. Drain off fat. Stir in undrained tomatoes, tomato paste, sugar, oregano, and garlic salt. Bring to boil and set aside. Spread cottage cheese over spaghetti crust. Fill with meat mixture. Bake uncovered 350° F. oven for 20 minutes. Sprinkle pie with mozzarella cheese. Bake an additional 5 minutes or until cheese is melted.

From the kitchen of Paula H.

Sensational Spaghetti

Medium onion, diced (about ½ c.)
2 cloves garlic, minced
¼ c. butter
1 tbsp. olive oil
½ lb. ground beef
½ lb. ground pork
½ lb. ground veal
½ green bell pepper, chopped
½ lb. mushrooms, chopped
2 6-oz. can tomato paste
28 oz. can stewed Italian
    tomatoes
1½ tsp. Worcestershire sauce
1½ tsp. angostura bitters
1 tbsp. sugar
½ c. dry red wine
½ tsp. salt
¼ tsp. freshly ground black
    pepper
½ tsp. celery salt
2 bay leaves
Dash of cayenne pepper
1 lb. spaghetti, cooked al dente
    and drained
Freshly grated Parmesan cheese

In large, heavy kettle, sauté onion

and garlic in butter and oil until transparent. Add beef, pork and veal, and brown over med. heat. Add green pepper, mushrooms, tomato paste, tomatoes, Worcestershire, bitters, sugar, wine, salt, pepper, celery salt, bay leaves and cayenne pepper. Simmer over low heat for 3 hours. Divide warm spaghetti among warmed individual plates and top with sauce. Sprinkle with Parmesan and serve immediately. Serves 6-8 main dish servings. From the kitchen of Catherine G.

Leave It Alone

 Don't wake up one morning and say, "Well, I'm feeling much stronger now, I think I can handle it from here."   Why do you think you are feeling stronger now? It's simple.   You gave Me your burdens and I'm taking care of them. I also renew your strength and cover you in my peace. Don't you know that if I give you these problems back, you will be right back where you started? Leave them with Me and forget about them. Just let Me do my job.   Author Unknown.

Microwave Ham and Broccoli Casserole

2 pkg. (8 oz.) frozen broccoli spears
2 c. cooked ham, cut in ½ in. cubes
Can (3 oz.) French fried onion rings
1 c. cheddar cheese, shredded
Can (10 ¾ oz.) cream of mushroom soup
¼ c. milk

Place both broccoli pkgs. in microwave and cook on HI for 6 minutes. Drain broccoli well, and remove from boxes. Arrange in 13-inch x 9-inch dish, alternating heads and stems. Top with ham, half the onion rings and cheese. Blend soup and milk. Pour over casserole.   Cover with wax paper. Microwave on HI for 8 to 10 minutes, or until broccoli stems are tender crisp. Sprinkle with remaining onion rings. Microwave uncovered, 5 to 6 minutes or until casserole is heated through. From the kitchen of Linda A.

Deep Dish Ham Pie

¼ cup butter or margarine
¼ cup flour
½ tsp. salt
¼ tsp. ground mustard
1/8 tsp. pepper
1 c. milk
1 tbsp. chopped onion
2½ c. cubed cooked ham
1 c. frozen peas, thawed
2 hard-cooked eggs, chopped
Pastry for single pie crust
Melt butter in pan, stir in flour, salt, mustard and pepper until smooth. Gradually add milk and onion, bring to boil. Cook and stir for 2 minutes or until thickened. Stir in ham, peas and eggs. Pour into an un-greased 9-inch pie plate. Place pie pastry over top and crimp edges. Cut 5-6 slits in top of crust. Bake at 425° F for 25 minutes or until crust is lightly brown.
From the kitchen of June T.

Baked Pork Chops

6 pork chops
¼ c. ketchup
¼ c. water
2 tsp. lemon juice
1 tsp. Worcestershire sauce
½ tsp. dry mustard
Small onion, sliced
Combine catsup, water, lemon juice, Worcestershire sauce and mustard. Pour over chops. Top with onion slices. Cover and bake in 350° F. oven for 1 hour or until done.
From the kitchen of Patsy S.

Spanish Pork Chops

4 pork chops
Salt and pepper
4 slices of onion
4 tbsp. ketchup
½ c. diluted vinegar or sweet pickle juice
Place pork chops in pan. Sprinkle lightly with salt and pepper. Place a slice of onion on each chop. Top with ketchup. Pour vinegar or pickle juice around the chops. Bake 1 hour at 350° F.
From the kitchen of Imodean D.

Foiled Pork Chops

For each serving:
Lean center-cut pork chop (5 oz.)
2 tbsp. unsweetened peach puree
    (baby food)
2 tsp. soy sauce
Optional: pinch of minced garlic
    (fresh or dried)
Optional: 2 tsp. onion flakes
¼ tsp. ground ginger

Trim and discard fringe fat from chops, set chops aside. Tear off square of aluminum foil for each chop. Combine remaining ingredients in the center of the foil. Turn the chop on the mixture to coat it well. Fold foil over chop. Arrange packets on a cookie tin and bake in a preheated 350° F. oven 1 hour or more, until tender. Open packets during last 15 minutes to permit chops to brown. Each serving has approximately 185 calories. You can even make up several packets at once and freeze the extras for baking later. (Increase baking time by 20 to 30 minutes when baking frozen packets.)
From the kitchen of June T.

Hungarian Sausage Loaf

1 c. dried mushroom
2 tbsp. butter
1 egg, beaten
1 lb of sausage
2 c. dry bread crumbs
1 tsp. paprika

Sauté mushrooms in butter. Combine mushrooms, egg, bread crumbs, and shape into loaf. Sprinkle with paprika. Place in pans. Bake covered 30 minutes at 350° F. Remove cover and bake for 30 more.
From the kitchen of Imodean D.

Bountiful Brunch Pizza

Crust:
Pkg. (24 oz.) frozen shredded
    hash brown patties, thawed
    and broken apart
1 egg, beaten with salt and pepper
    to taste

Preheat oven to 400° F. Combine hash browns, egg, salt and pepper well. Spread potato mixture into a 14 inch circle on a baking pan or pizza pan. Pat down to firm crust. Bake for 20 minutes. Remove from oven and add your favorite toppings. Return to oven for 10 more minutes.

Toppings:

7 eggs

½ c. milk

salt and pepper to taste

Wisk eggs and milk together. Season with salt and pepper. Cook in pan or microwave to make scrambled eggs. Put scrambled eggs on crust as first layer then add the following toppings:

1 c. chopped ham

½ c. sliced mushrooms and ¼ c. green onion slices

¼ c. chopped green bell pepper

1½ c. (6 oz.) shredded cheddar cheese

Remember: Return to oven for 10 more minutes

From the kitchen of Alecia M.

Make promises sparingly and keep them faithfully, no matter what the cost.

Tilapia Fish

Lightly flour, salt and pepper thawed out fillets.

Brown about 5-7 minutes on each side in small amount of canola oil.

Drain oil. Dot with butter and lemon juice. (Wal-Mart Flash Frozen Individually Fillets - package is about 4 for $3.47.)

From the kitchen of Paula H.

Microwave Sole in Lemon Parsley Butter

½ c. butter or margarine

2 tbsp. corn starch

3 tbsp. lemon

1 tsp. dried parsley flakes

1/8 tsp. celery salt

Dash of pepper

2 lb. frozen sole fillets, thawed

Place butter in 2 quart (11-inch x 7-inch) glass baking dish. Microwave on 'Roast' for about 2 minutes or until melted. Blend in cornstarch, lemon juice, parsley, celery salt and pepper. Arrange fillets with thick edges toward outside of dish. Cover with wax paper. Microwave on HI for 8-9 minutes or until fillets flake easily. Let stand, covered 5 minutes before serving. About 6 servings.

From the kitchen of Linda A.

Spanish Rice

4 slices bacon
½ tsp. salt
1 c. onion, chopped
¼ c. green pepper, chopped
2 - 10½ or 11 oz. cans tomato
    soup
½ c. rice
½ c. water
4 whole cloves
Bay leaf
Cut bacon in small pieces. Fry until crisp and remove bacon. Cook onion and green pepper in bacon fat. Drain fat. Add all other ingredients. Cover lightly and cook slowly 50 minutes. Stir occasionally. Remove cloves and bay leaf; sprinkle crisp bacon over the top and serve.
From the kitchen of Imodean D.

Nothing else ruins the truth like stretching it.
Compassion is difficult to give away because it keeps coming back.

Spanish Rice

1 c. rice
3 tbsp. oil
10 ½ oz. chicken broth
Medium onion, chopped
Garlic clove
1½ c. canned tomatoes (1 can)
1 tsp. cumin
Salt and pepper
Brown rice. Stir in remaining ingredients. Cover. Cook slowly about 25 minute.
From the kitchen of Paula H.

Homemade Noodles

1½ c. flour
3 tbsp. water
1 tsp. salt
Egg
1 tsp. fat
Mix to form a stiff dough. Divide into three parts and roll each as thin as possible and cut into strips.
From the kitchen of Imodean D.

He who angers you controls you.
Worry is the darkroom in which negatives can develop.

Egg Souffle

Slices of Whole Wheat or 12 grain bread to line the bottom of the casserole

8 eggs, slightly beaten (more if desired)

4 c. milk

1 lb. or less cheddar cheese (sharp) grated,

1 lb. lean sausage (Jimmy Dean) cooked and drained

½ tsp. or less salt, if desired

½ tsp. pepper

2 tsp. dry mustard

Place slices of bread in 9-inch x 13-inch greased casserole dish. Push and get in as much bread as is possible. Cut partial slices to completely cover the bottom. Put cooked crumbled sausage on top of bread. Whisk eggs, milk, salt, pepper and dry mustard together and pour over the bread and sausage. Sprinkle cheese on top. Place in the refrigerator overnight. Bake at 350° F for 45 minutes. Let stand 8-10 minutes before serving.

From the kitchen of Linda A.

Best Sermons are Lived Not Preached

Today, I interviewed my grandmother for part of a research paper I'm working on for my Psychology class. When I asked her to define success in her own words, she said, "Success is when you look back at your life and the memories make you smile."

Today, I asked my mentor - a very successful business man in his 70s- what his top 3 tips are for success. He smiled and said, "Read something no one else is reading, think something no one else is thinking, and do something no one

else is doing."

Today, after a 72 hour shift at the fire station, a woman ran up to me at the grocery store and gave me a hug. When I tensed up, she realized I didn't recognize her. She let go with tears of joy in her eyes and the most sincere smile and said, "On 9-11-2001, you carried me out of the World Trade Center."

Today, a boy in a wheelchair saw me desperately struggling on crutches with my broken leg and offered to carry my backpack and books for me. He helped me all the way across campus to my class and as he was leaving he said, "I hope you feel better soon."

Today, I was feeling down because the results of a biopsy came back malignant. When I got home, I opened an e-mail that said, "Thinking of you today. If you need me, I'm just a phone call away." It was from a high school friend I hadn't seen in 30 years. Author Unknown

Talk To Me

I want you to forget a lot of things. Forget what was making you crazy. Forget the worry and the fretting because you know I'm in control. But there's one thing I pray you never forget.

Please, don't forget to talk to Me - OFTEN! I love YOU! I want to hear your voice. I want you to include Me in on the things going on in your life. I want to hear you talk about your friends and family. Prayer is simply you having a conversation with Me. I want to be your dearest friend.

Author Unknown

Chapter 9

Pies

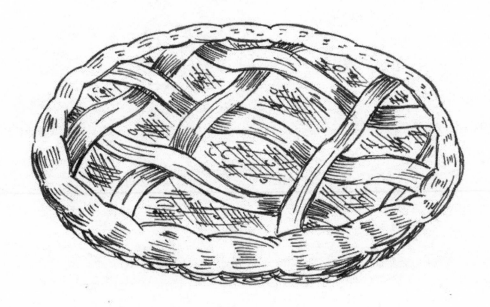

Index of Pie Recipes

Pie Crust

6 tbsp. butter melted in pie pan
½ tsp. salt
1 c. sifted flour
1 tbsp. water

Mix well in a pie pan, spreading it with your fingers around the pan. Bake as usual.

From kitchen of Phyliss T.

Pie Crust

5 c. flour, sifted
2 tsp. salt
½ tsp. baking powder
1 tbsp. sugar
1¾ c. shortening
2 egg yolks

Mix flour, salt, sugar, and baking powder. Add in the shortening. Put the two egg yolks in the bottom of a measuring cup and beat with a fork. Add enough water to make 7/8 cups of liquid. Mix in well with the other ingredients. Makes five pie crusts.

From the kitchen of Evelyn B.

Frozen Pie Crust

Bag (5 lb.) flour
2 tbsp. salt
Can (3 lb.) shortening
1 c. white corn syrup
3 c. cold water

In a large bowl, mix flour and salt well. With an electric mixer, cut in shortening until mixture resembles coarse crumbs. Stir in corn syrup and water. Divide dough into fist-size balls. Place into individual bags, then into a large re-sealable bag. Freeze. Remove 1 ball for each crust that you need. Let thaw 1 hour at room temperature or overnight in refrigerator before rolling out. Dough will be soft, and you can refreeze unused dough. Yields 21 to 22 single pie crust.

From the kitchen of Evelyn B.

Don't wait for six strong men to take you to church.

Fresh Strawberry Pie

1 1/3 c. sugar
1 c. water
¼ c. cornstarch
¼ c. water
⅛ tsp. salt
1 tbsp. lemon juice
16 oz. fresh strawberries, sliced
Red food coloring
Whipped cream
Baked pie shell

Mix water and sugar. Boil to melt sugar. Add cornstarch mixed with ¼ c. water to syrup. Cook slowly, 10-15 minutes or until clear. Add salt, lemon juice and food coloring. Let cool - then add strawberries and pour into baked pie shell. (If using fresh peaches, add 1 tablespoon butter to hot liquid.) Add 1 tablespoon water mixed well in a pie pan, spreading it with your finders around the pan. Bake as usual.

From kitchen of unknown

Mother's No Cook Strawberry Pie

1½ c. fine vanilla wafer crumbs, hold out 2 tablespoons
2/3 c. melted butter
½ c. room temperature margarine
1½ c. sifted powdered sugar
2 eggs beaten
1 tsp. vanilla
1½ c. drained sweetened strawberry slices (fresh or frozen)
2 c. heavy whipped cream
¼ c. sugar

Mix 1¼ cups of wafer crumbs with melted butter. Press into buttered 9 inch pie pan and chill until firm. Cream oleo and powdered sugar. Add beaten eggs and vanilla, beating until fluffy. Pour into crust. Whip cream into soft peaks gradually adding ¼ cup sugar and beating into stuff peaks. Fold strawberries (if frozen strawberries are used, thaw and drain first) into whipped cream and spread over first mixture in the crust. Sprinkle with 2 tbsp of crumbs. Refrigerate until firm, about 8 hours.

From the kitchen of Irene T.

Aunt Thel's Strawberry Pie

Pkg. strawberries, cut up
1 c. sugar
2 egg whites, beaten
1 tbsp. lemon juice
½ c. whipping cream, whipped
1 tsp. vanilla

Beat the egg whites until stiff, gradually add sugar, strawberries, and lemon juice. (about 15 minutes) Fold the strawberries, whipped cream and vanilla into the first group of ingredients. Put in baked pie shell. Put in freezer for ½ day or overnight.
From the kitchen of Thel H.

Strawberry Pie

Baked 9-in. crust
1½ qt. strawberries
1 c. sugar
¼ tsp. salt
¼ c. cornstarch
1 c. water
Red food coloring
1 c. whipped cream or whipped topping
Crush ½-quart of strawberries; add sugar, salt, cornstarch, water and food coloring. Cook until thick and clear. Heap 1 quart strawberries in baked crust. Allow the cooked mixture to cool. When cool, pour over berries in crust. Chill. Top with whipped topping. Refrigerate.
From the kitchen of June T.

Monarch Cherry Pie

Can cherries
2/3 c. sugar
1½ tbsp. corn starch
1 tbsp. butter
⅛ tsp. salt
¼ tsp. almond extract
Put cherries in a pie shell. Mix corn starch, salt, and sugar. Pour over cherries. Mix in juice and extract.   Dot with butter.
From the kitchen of Catherine G.

"Make yourself at home, clean my kitchen!"

Pineapple Chiffon Pie

Can crushed pineapple
Envelope un-flavored gelatin
1 c. pineapple juice
1 tbsp. lemon
½ c. water
¼ tsp. salt
¾ c. sugar (½ c. + ¼ c.)
3 eggs, separated
1 tsp. grated lemon rind
Drain pineapple reserving both juice and pineapple.   Dissolve gelatin in ¼ cup of the pineapple juice.   Combine remaining juice, lemon juice, water, salt and ½ cup sugar, and bring to a boil.   Stir in softened gel. Stir until dissolved. Separate yolks and whites of the egg and save the yolk   Beat the egg yolks. Add a little hot mixture to the egg yolks, beating well to keep the egg yolks from premature cooking. Add remaining hot mixture, stirring constantly.   Cook over low heat for 3 minutes, stirring constantly. Chill until thickened.   Stir in grated lemon rind and ½ cup crushed pineapple. Beat egg whites and
¼ cup sugar until stiff.   Fold gelatin mixture into egg whites.

Pour into baked pie shell.   Chill until firm.   May decorate with whipped cream and remaining crushed pineapple.
From the kitchen of Thel H.

Hawaiian Pie

4 eggs, well beaten
2 c. sugar
1 tbsp. flour
Small can crushed pineapple
Can angel flake coconut
Stick of oleo or margarine
1 tsp. vanilla
1 tbsp. corn meal
Mix all together. Put in an unbaked pie shell. Bake in a slow oven at 350° F. or 325° F. about 30 minutes.
From the kitchen of Phyliss T.

Six Best Doctors in the World

1. Sunlight
2. Rest
3. Exercise
4. Diet
5. Self Confidence
6. Friends

Maintain them in all stages of Life and enjoy a Healthy life.

Cherry Cream Cheese Pie

Filling:

8 oz. pkg. cream cheese and
15 oz. can sweetened condensed
   milk
1/3 c. lemon juice
1 tsp. vanilla

Blend cream cheese, sweetened condensed milk, lemon juice and vanilla. Pour into a pressed graham cracker crust. Chill. Make cherry glaze and spread over the top. Chill for at least 12 hours before serving.

Graham Cracker Crust:

1¼ c. graham cracker crumbs
2/3 stick margarine, melted
3 tbsp. confectioners' sugar

Combine and press into pie pan. Chill

Cherry Glaze:

½ c. cherry juice, drained
2 tbsp. sugar
2 tbsp. cornstarch
red food coloring
Can of cherries, drained

Cook first three ingredients until thickened. Add a few drops of red food coloring and cherries. Garnish top of pie.

From the kitchen of Paula H.

Fresh Peach Pie

Baked 9 in. pie crust
⅛ oz. pkg. cream cheese
2 c. powdered sugar & 1/3 c. sugar
1 small carton of half and half

Combine cheese and powdered sugar. Beat with mixer until smooth. Spread mixture on pie crust. Peel and slice peaches to fill rest of pie shell and put peaches on creamed filling. Whip the half and half, sweeten with sugar, as desired, and spread over the top of the peaches. Slice and enjoy.

From the kitchen of June T.

Peach Cobbler

1 c. sugar and 1 c. flour
1 tsp. baking powder
¼ tsp. salt
½ pt. whipping cream, not
   whipped
3 tbsp. melted butter
2 c. fruit

Mix the sugar, flour, baking powder and salt. Add the whipped cream and stir. Pour into 8 x 8-inch melted butter coated pan. Add fruit last. Bake at 375° for 45 minutes.

From the kitchen of Mrs. Baker

Peach Custard Pie

2 eggs, beaten
¾ c. milk
2 tbsp. [heaping] cornstarch
3 c. sliced peaches
⅓ c. sugar
Mix eggs, milk and cornstarch.
Add sugar to sliced peaches. Put
peaches in unbaked pie crust.
Cover peaches with egg-milk-
cornstarch mixture. You may
need a little more milk or peaches
for a deep dish. For smaller dish,
cut down. Bake 425° F. for 15
minutes and then 350° F. for 30
minutes or until knife comes out
clean.
From the kitchen of June T.

Essie's Cobbler

¼ c. butter
½ c. sugar
1 tsp. vanilla
1 c. flour
2 tsp. baking powder
¼ tsp. salt
½ c. milk
drained fruit
¼ to ½ c. sugar
1 c. fruit juice
Heat oven to 375° F. Cream

butter and sugar. Stir in sifted
ingredients and milk. Pour into
loaf pan. Spoon fruit and batter.
Sprinkle with sugar. Bake 45-50
minutes.
From the kitchen of Susan M.

Sugarless Apple Pie

8 oz. pure unsweetened apple juice
1½ tbsp. cornstarch
1 tsp. cinnamon and 1 tsp. nutmeg
2 tbsp. butter or margarine
4 Golden Delicious apples, peeled,
    cored and sliced (may add ½ c.
    raisins to apples)
2 pie crusts
In a small saucepan, bring 6 oz. of
the apple juice to boil. Mix
cornstarch with remaining 2 oz. of
juice till smooth and add to the
boiling juice with the spices and
butter. Heat and stir till very
thick. Remove from the heat.
Place apples in bottom crust.
Pour juice mixture over apples.
Top with second crust, putting a
few slits in the top. Bake at 350°
F. for an hour.
From the kitchen of Cheryl B.

Old Fashioned Fried Pies

2 c. flour

1 tsp. salt

1/3 c. shortening

Ice water

Filling recipe below

Stir together flour and salt.

Cut shortening into flour mixture until crumbs are the size of small peas.

Gradually add water (about a cup) to make a soft dough. Roll out ¼ inch thickness on a lightly floured pastry cloth. Cut in five inch rounds (use a sharp pointed knife and a card board cut out from the top of a coffee can.) Put 1½ tablespoon filling on half of each circle, keeping it ½ inch form the edge. Seal edges. Fry in oil at 360° F, 2-3 minutes, frying to a light brown. Drain on paper towels. Dust with powdered sugar if desired. They are veryyyyyy gggggoooooddd to eat warm. They may be frozen. Makes 10 -12 fried pies.

From the kitchen of Irene T.

Fried Pie Filling

1 lb. dried fruit (apricots, apples, peaches, cherries, blue berries, cranberries, etc.)

1 c. sugar

1½ c. water

If apricots are very dry, soak in water, for a few hours up to overnight. Cook the apricots and water until thick. Add sugar and continue cooking until sugar is melted. Cool to luke warm.

Other dried fruit may be used with this same recipe.

From the kitchen of Irene T.

Are You Connected

God has no BLACKBERRY but he's my favorite contact.

He is not on FACEBOOK but he is my best friend.

He is not on TWITTER but I still follow Him, and even without the INTERNET I am always connected to him.

He has no a GMAIL account but he's always online.

Author Unknown

Mother's Fried Pies

2 c. flour
2 tsp. baking powder
½ tsp. salt
2 tbsp. shortening
¾ c. milk
Cooked fruit
Sift flour, baking powder and salt. Cut in shortening. Add milk gradually. Knead lightly on floured surface. Roll ¼ in. and cut round size of saucer. Place 1 tbsp. cooked fruit on ½ of pastry. Fold. Moisten inner edges with cold water and press together with a fork. Prick top several times. Brown in skillet. Turn several times. Remove. Drain on paper towels.
Filling: Cook in a skillet of shallow oil - water and sugar with fruit of choice, apricots, cherries, etc.
From the kitchen of Paula H.

In the sentence of life, the devil may be a comma--but never let him be the period.

Fried Pies from Dixie

2 c. flour
2 tsp. baking powder
½ tsp. salt
3 tbsp. shortening
¾ c. milk
Cooked fruit
Sift flour before measuring, then sift with baking powder and salt. Cut shortening into flour mixture. Add milk gradually, mixing into dry ingredients. Toss into floured bread board, knead lightly. Roll out about ¼ in. thick and cut in rounds about size of saucer. Place cooked fruit: raisins, apricot, apple sauce or any canned fruit drained or cherry pie filling and put one tablespoon of fruit on dough, moisten outer edge of crust and fold over and press together with tongs of fork. Prick top several times and brown and in shallow fat in skillet. Turn several times and place on a soft paper towel to drain.
From the kitchen of Irene T.

It's the door

Thought I would share this with those who might, occasionally, have the same problem.

Ever walk into a room with some purpose in mind, only to completely forget what that purpose was? Turns out, doors themselves are to blame for these strange memory lapses.

Psychologists at the University of Notre Dame have discovered that passing through a doorway triggers what's known as an event boundary in the mind, separating one set of thoughts and memories from the next.

Your brain files away the thoughts you had in the previous room and prepares a blank slate for the new locale. So it's not aging, it's the stupid door! Thank goodness for scientific studies like this!

Author unknown

Chocolate Pies

(For 2 pies)

2 heaping tbsp. cocoa
2½ c. sugar
6 tbsp. flour
½ tsp. salt
3 c. milk
5 eggs (separate yolks and whites)
2 tbsp. butter or oleo
1 tsp. vanilla
½ tsp. cream of tartar
2 baked pie shells

Sift together cocoa, flour, salt and 2½ cups sugar. Add milk and stir well. Cook until it thickens good. Take off heat and add well beaten egg yolks. (Pour a little hot mixture in the egg yolks stirring constantly.) Then pour rest into hot mix slowly, while stirring. Cook until medium thick then add butter or oleo and vanilla. Cool. Pour into baked pie shell. Whip egg whites, with cream of tartar until foamy. Then add 10 tablespoons (½ cup + 2 tablespoons) sugar, beating until merangue.

From the kitchen of Mrs. Reece

Chocolate Mousse Pies

Meringue Crusts:

4 egg whites
½ tsp. vanilla
1/8 tsp. salt
1 c. sugar
¼ tsp. cream of tartar
c. pecans, chopped

Combine egg whites, vanilla, salt and cream of tartar. Beat stiff. Add sugar gradually, beating until very stiff and sugar is dissolved. Sprinkle the pecans in the bottom for two well-greased 8 inch pie pans. Spread the ingredient mixture over the pecans. Build up the sides. Bake at 257° F. for one hour. Cool, fill with filling.

Filling:

1- 9 oz. pkg. semi-sweet chocolate chips (1½ c.)
Egg
3 egg yolks
1½ tsp. vanilla
3 egg whites
1½ c. heavy cream, whipped

Melt chocolate chips over hot, not boiling water. Remove from the water. Beat in the egg, and yolks one at a time. Add vanilla. Beat whites until they form peaks when beater is raised. Fold in cream, whipped and chocolate mixture. Divide the mixture between the two pie shells. Refrigerate until well chilled. (12-24 hours) This is very important. If not refrigerated long enough, crusts will be tough. To serve, top with one cup heavy cream, whipped, which has been sweetened to taste.

From the kitchen of Catherine G.

Chocolate Pie Filling (2 pies)

1½ c. sugar
½ c. flour
¼ c. cocoa
6 egg yolks
3 ¾ - 4 c. milk
2 tbsp. butter
2 tsp. vanilla
1 pie crust, baked

Mix sugar, flour and cocoa in a sauce pan. Add milk and egg yolks and mix with a wire whip. Cook until mixture bubbles. Add butter and vanilla. Put mixture into two pie crust.

From the kitchen of Catherine G.

Chocolate Nut Pie

1 tbsp. Knox Gelatin
¼ c. cold water
Pkg. semi-sweet chocolate
⅔ c. sugar
2 eggs
½ tsp. vanilla
½ c. nuts, chopped
1 c. dream whip
Melt gelatin in cold water. Melt semi-sweet chocolate over low heat. Take off the burner and stir in the gelatin till smooth. Beat sugar in eggs till the sugar is dissolved. Then add to the chocolate mixture and stir well. Add vanilla and nuts. Refrigerate till mixture starts to thicken, then add dream whip and chill thoroughly. It is supposed to be put in a baked pie shell. When one does not feel like making the crust put in individual sherbet dishes.
From the kitchen of Marjorie S.

"I'm on a 30 day diet; so far I have lost 15 days."

Chocolate Pecan Pie

Stick butter, melted
1 c. sugar
2 eggs
½ c. flour
1 tsp. vanilla
1 c. chopped pecans
1 c. chocolate chips
Unbaked pie shell
Add melted butter to sugar, and cream well. Add eggs, one at a time, and beat after the last. Stir in the flour, vanilla, and pecans, mix well. Cover bottom of pie shell with chocolate chips. Pour mixture over the chocolate chips. Bake at 350° F. and for 40 - 45 minutes. Better served warm. Freezes well.
From the kitchen of Bonnie S.

Sign at a reducing salon: "24 Shaping Days until Christmas."

Mother's Pecan Pie

1 c. white Karo
¾ c. sugar
¼ tsp. salt
1 tsp. vanilla
¼ c. melted butter
3 eggs slightly beaten
1 c. pecans

Mix and pour into a 9-inch pastry shell, uncooked. Bake at 425° F for 10 minutes. Then turn down oven and bake at 325° F for an additional 35-40 minutes.

From the kitchen of Catherine G.

Pecan Pie

3 tbsp. flour
1½ c. sugar
4 eggs
3/8 c. corn syrup
1 c. pecans, halves or chopped

Mix the flour and sugar. Beat the eggs and stir eggs and syrup into the dry ingredients. Add the pecans. Pour the mixture into un-baked pie shell and bake at 325° F. for ½ hour or until set.

From the kitchen of Mattie H. and Irene T.

Magic Lemon Pie

Can (14oz.) Eagle Brand Sweetened condensed milk
½ c. lemon juice
1 tsp. grated lemon rind
2 eggs, separated
8 or 9 in. prepared graham cracker pie crust
¼ tsp. cream of tartar
4 tbsp. sugar

Preheat oven to 325° F. In a medium bowl combine: eagle brand, lemon juice, and egg yolks; stir mixture until it thickens. Pour into chilled graham cracker crust. For topping you can use cool whip and refrigerate or make meringue. For meringue; in medium bowl beat egg whites and cream of tartar on high speed until soft peaks form. Gradually beat in sugar on medium speed, one tablespoon at a time; beat four minutes longer or until sugar is dissolved and stiff gloss peaks form. Spread meringue over pie, carefully sealing to edge of crust to prevent shrinking. Bake 12 to 15 minutes or until meringue is lightly browned. Cool and refrigerate.

From the kitchen of Susanne T.

Buttermilk Pie

5 eggs, well beaten
1 c. buttermilk
3 c. sugar
3 tbsp. Flour
1 stick oleo or butter
1 tsp. lemon extract
1 tsp. vanilla
2 un-baked 9 in. pie shells
Combine and pour into pie shells and bake at 350° F. until firm, about 50-60 minutes.
From the kitchen of Thel H.

Buttermilk Pie

3¾ c. sugar
½ c. flour
½ tsp. salt
6 eggs
1 c. buttermilk
2 sticks margarine, melted
1 tsp. vanilla
1 tsp. butter flavoring
2 unbaked pie crusts, 9 in.
Blend sugar, flour, salt, and eggs. Add buttermilk and vanilla. Don't beat. Gently stir in two sticks melted margarine and butter flavoring. Pour in pie crusts and bake at 350° F. for 50-60 minutes.
From the kitchen of Paula H.

Delightful Pumpkin Pie

1½ c. pumpkin
⅔ c. brown sugar
1 tsp. cinnamon
½ tsp. ginger
1 tsp. salt
2 eggs
2 c. milk
Combine ingredients and turn into unbaked pastry shell and bake at a high temperature at first at 450° F. to cook bottom and continue cooking at 325° F. until a silver knife come out clean. Do not let pie fail as that makes it watery. Top pie with a drizzle of honey and whipped cream.
From the kitchen of Ethel A.

The brightest future will always be based on a forgotten past; you can't go forward in life until you let go of your past failures and heartaches.

.

Coconut Box Pie

(Bulk)

3 pie shells
2 qt. coffee cream
6 eggs
6 oz. corn starch
1 lb. 4 oz. sugar
When mixed, bring to a boil.
Remove from the stove and cool
down by setting the sauce pan in a
sink of cold water, stirring to start
cooling down. Add vanilla and
continue stirring. Then pour into
pie shells and refrigerate. Add
whipped cream when serving.
From the Skirvin Tower Hotel,
Oklahoma City, OK, 1960.

Accept the fact that some days
you're the pigeon, and some days
you're the statue!

Always keep your words soft
and sweet, just in case you have to
eat them.

Always read stuff that will
make you look good if you die in
the middle of it.

If you can't be kind, at least
have the decency to be vague.
Author Unknown

for a
the c   was able
to have him fitted for a set of
hearing aids that allowed the
gentleman to hear 100%

The elderly gentleman went
back in a month to the doctor and
the doctor said, "Your hearing is
perfect. Your family must be
really pleased that you can hear
again."

The gentleman replied, "Oh, I
haven't told my family yet. I just
sit around and listen to the
conversations. I've changed my
will three times!"
Author Unknown

ght Things to Remember

eople in this world love you so much they would die for you.

15 people in this world love you in some way.

night, SOMEONE thinks about you before they go to sleep.

u mean the world to someone.

If not for you, someone may not be living.

6. When you make the biggest mistake ever, something good can still come from it.

7. When you think the world has turned its back on you, take a look: you most likely turned your back on the world.

8. Always remember the compliments you received. Forget about the rude remarks.

Trust Me

Once you've given your burdens to Me, quit trying to take them back. Trust in Me. Have the faith that I will take care of all your needs, your problems and your trials. Problems with the kids? Put them on My list. Problem with finances? Put it on My list. Problems with your emotional roller coaster? For My sake, put it on My list. I want to help you. All you have to do is ask.

Arthur Unknown

When one door closes, God opens two

Chapter 9
Cookies and Such

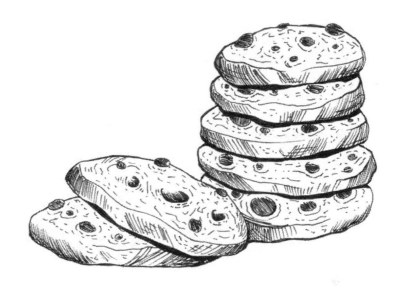

Index of Cookie and Such Recipes

Apple Kugel

Can apple pie filling
¾ c. flour
¾ c. sugar
Combine and place in large pie pan or
8-inch x 8-inch pan. Add topping of crushed corn flake crumbs.
Bake at 350° F for 1 hour.
From the Kitchen of Michou A.

Peanut Butter Balls

1 c. peanut butter
4 c. Rice Krispies
2 sticks oleo (soft) or use butter
1 lb. powdered sugar
Mix together and roll into walnut sized balls. Mixture may be gooey.
Dip in dipping chocolate and place on waxed paper.
From the kitchen of Barbara U.

Chewy Peanut Balls

1 c. peanut butter
1 c. honey OR ½ c. molasses + ½ c. corn syrup OR ½ c. dark syrup + ½. Honey OR 1 c. any mixture that suits you.
2 c. dry milk

Mix all ingredients well. Roll in high-protein
cereal crumbs. Chill in refrigerator.
From the kitchen of Linda A.

Peanut Butter Cookies

1 c. white sugar and
1 c. brown sugar
1 c. peanut butter
1 c. Crisco
2 eggs
1 tbsp. water
1 tsp. vanilla
2½ c. flour
½ tsp. baking soda
½ tsp. salt
Cream sugars, peanut butter and Crisco. Beat in eggs, water and vanilla. Sift together flour, salt and baking soda and add to mixture. Make into balls lay out on a cookie sheet and mash each one with a fork.   Bake at 350° F. for about 8 minutes. Put on paper towels to cool before storing in a container.
From the kitchen of Irene T.

Peanut Butter Molasses Squares

1½ c. flour
1½ tsp. baking powder
½ tsp. soda
1 tsp. cinnamon
½ tsp. cloves
½ tsp. salt
⅓ c. soft shortening
½ c. peanut butter
½ c. sugar
1 egg
½ c. light molasses
½ c. hot water
½ c. finely chopped peanuts

Heat oven 350° F. Grease a 12-inch x 9-inch x 2-inch pan lined with wax paper and grease and flour paper. Sift together dry ingredients. Work shortening and peanut butter into bowl until creamy. Add sugar and beat well. Add egg and molasses. Beat until blended. Add hot water or coffee alternately with dry ingredients to creamed mixture. Mix well after each addition. Pour into pan sprinkled with nuts. Bake for 30 or 35 minutes. Cool slightly and remove from pan to wire rack. Cool and cut into 1⅜ x 2⅜ inch bars. Makes 30 bars.
From the kitchen of Ethel A.

Mother's Christmas Angel Wings

1 c. chopped dates
Stick of oleo
¾ c. sugar

Bring to a boil. Simmer for 5 minutes. Remove from heat.
Add/Stir in:
3 c. Rice Krispies
1 c. nuts
15 Maraschino cherries, chopped

Form into balls. Leave loose, not to firm. Roll in cocoanut. Serve.
From the kitchen of Irene T.

Peanut Patties

3 c. sugar
1 c. white syrup
1 c. Milnot
3 c. raw peanuts
Food coloring

Cook until soft ball stage then beat. Then add:
1 tsp. vanilla
1½ - 2 tsp. butter

Drop by tablespoon on wax paper.
From the kitchen of Imodean D.

Wilma's Angel Cookies

½ c. butter or margarine
½ c. shortening
½ c. brown sugar
½ c. white sugar
1 egg
1 tsp. soda
1 tsp. cream or tarter
1 tsp. vanilla
½ tsp. salt
2 c. flour

Cream butter and shortening. Add sugar and egg and cream. Sift dry ingredients and add to mixture. Roll into small balls. (will be sticky) Dip in water and then sugar. Place, sugar side up, on greased cookie sheets. Bake at 375° F. for 6-10 minutes or until done.

From the kitchen of Wilma V.

Mother's Snowballs

1 c. butter or oleo
2 c. ground pecans
2 c. flour
¼ c. sugar

Beat oleo until creamy. Add remaining ingredients. Beat. Roll into balls. Bake on ungreased cookie sheet in a 300° F oven for 40 minutes. Roll in confectioners' sugar while warm. Cool. Then roll again. Makes 4 dozen.

From the kitchen of Irene T.

Blonde Brownie

2 c. flour
1 tsp. baking powder
¼ tsp. baking soda
1 tsp. salt
1 c. margarine or butter
2 c. brown sugar
2 eggs, lightly beaten
2 tsp. vanilla
1 c. chopped pecans
12 oz. pkg. semi-sweet chocolate pieces.

Melt butter in saucepan. Stir in brown sugar. Pour into large bowl. Cool. Stir in eggs and vanilla and dry ingredients. Stir in the pecans and two-thirds of the chocolate pieces. Pour batter into greased, oblong pan. Sprinkle batter with remaining chocolate pieces, pressing down slightly. Bake at 350° F. for 30 minutes, or until mixture pulls away from the edge of pan. Cool in pan. Cut into squares.

From the kitchen of Paula H.

Melba's Brownies

2 heaping tbsp. cocoa
2/3 c. shortening (use oil)
2 c. sugar
4 eggs
1½ c. flour
1 tsp. baking powder
½ tsp. salt
1 c. nuts, chopped
Powdered sugar
Melt shortening, cocoa and sugar.
Beat in the eggs. Stir in the flour,
baking powder, salt and nuts.
Bake at 350° F. for 30-31 minutes.
Sprinkle with powdered sugar.
From the kitchen of Paula H.

Brownies

(Bulk)

Cream together at low speed:
3 lb. sugar
1 lb. butter
10 eggs
Pound honey and 12 oz. cocoa
Add alternately until mixed:
Pint coffee creamer, dry
1½ lb. cake flour
Last add:
Little red coloring
shot of vanilla
1 lb. pecans
Bake at 350° F. For 35 minutes.

From the Skirvin Tower Hotel,
Oklahoma City, OK, 1960.

Brownie Mix

6 c. flour
4 tsp. baking powder
4 tsp. salt
8 c. sugar
2½ c. cocoa
2 c. shortening
2/3 c. nuts (optional)
Mix the dry ingredients together.
Cut in the shortening. Store in a
covered container.
To make brownies from mix:
2 c. brownie mix
2 eggs
1 tsp. vanilla
2 c. nuts (Optional)
Beat the eggs and add the vanilla
and brownie mix. Add the nuts.
Bake in a 8-inch by 8-inch pan for
25 minutes at 350° F.
For a larger amount:
3 c. brownie mix
3 eggs
1 tsp. vanilla
3 c. nuts (optional)
Mix as above. Bake in a greased
7 inch x 11 inch pan at 350°F. for
about 35 minutes.
Used in Expanded Nutrition

Program, Douglas County, Lawrence, Kansas by Linda A.

Carmel Nut Slices

(Refrigerator Cookies)

Cream:

1 c. shortening (part butter or margarine) or (½ c. oil and ½ c. butter or margarine)

2 c. brown sugar

2 eggs

Sift together and add to above:

3½ c. flour (or part whole wheat flour)

1 tsp. baking soda

½ tsp. salt

Mix in:

1 c. nuts

Make into 2 or 3 rolls 2 inches in diameter on wax paper. Wrap in wax paper. Chill overnight or freeze. Slice 1/8 inch thick slices as many as desired for the occasion. Place on an ungreased cookie sheet and bake at 400° F. for 8 to 10 minutes. Makes about 10 dozen.

From the kitchen of Wilma V.

Cherry Torte

Mix:

1½ c. sugar

1 c. flour and 1 tsp. soda

1 tsp. cinnamon

¼ tsp. salt

2 c. drained cherries (1 – No. 2 can)

3 eggs, beaten

3 tbsp. butter, melted

½ c. chopped nuts

Sift dry ingredients. Add eggs, cherries and melted butter. Bake in 350° F. oven for 45 minutes. Cut in squares and serve.

From the kitchen of Juanita H.

Lemon Fluff

Pkg. Lemon Jello

1 c. sugar and 1½ c. hot water

Can of Milnot, chilled and whipped

Can crushed pineapple

Juice of lemon and grated rind

Juice of drained pineapple

Combine jello, sugar, hot liquid and lemon. Chill and whip it. Mix whipped Milnot and drained pineapple. Pour into Pyrex pan, lined with vanilla wafers. Add crumbs of vanilla wafers on top and refrigerate.

From the kitchen of Kattie J.

Kohas Cookies

(Virginia's Coconut)

1 c. butter
1 c. sugar
½ lb. coconut
2 c. flour
1 egg
1 tsp. vanilla

Cream butter and sugar. Add egg and vanilla. Mix in the flour and then the coconut. Divide dough in half, roll in logs and refrigerate until cold. Cut into ¼ inch slices. Place on a cookie sheet and bake at 350° F. for 10-12 minutes.

From the kitchen of Virginia D.

Old friends are like Gold! New friends are Diamonds! If you get a Diamond, don't forget the Gold! Because to hold a Diamond, you always need a base of Gold.

Raisin and Bean Cookies

2 c. sugar (or 1 c. sugar and 1 c. stevia)
1½ tsp. vanilla
1 c. olive or canola oil (or use ½ c. oil and ½ c. applesauce)
2 tsp. cinnamon
1 c. powdered milk plus ⅓ c. more unsweetened applesauce
2 c. blended pinto beans plus 3 tbsp. liquid from beans, water or milk
3 eggs (or 6 egg whites)
1 c. applesauce
¼ tsp. salt
1 tsp. baking powder
1 tsp. baking soda
4 c. flour or (2 c. all purpose flour and 2 c. whole wheat flour)
2 c. raisins or dried cranberries
2 c. nuts (chopped)

Cream together oil, sugar, powdered milk and blended pinto beans. (You may want to put applesauce in blender with beans, to help in making a fairly smooth blend.) Add eggs, applesauce, and vanilla. Beat well. Sift all dry ingredients and blend into creamed mixture. Add raisins and nuts. Bake in two 1-inch deep jelly roll pans about 13-inch x 18-inch at 325°- 350° F. for about 18 to 20 minutes. You may have to bake 1 pan at a time according to the size of your oven. Cool. This is a soft nutritious sheet cookie to be cut into bars. Makes about 100 small bars. Flavor develops the second or third day. If not going to serve in 4 or 5 days, freeze the remaining cookies.

From the kitchen of Linda A.

Chocolate Chip Cookies

Cream:
⅔ c. Shortening
⅔ c. butter
1 c. sugar
1 c. brown sugar
Add:
2 eggs
2 tsp. vanilla
Combine these ingredients &
add:
3 c. flour
1 tsp. baking soda
1 tsp. salt
Add:
Bag chocolate chips
1 c. walnuts optional
Bake at 375° F for 8-10 minutes.
From the kitchen of Irene T.

Chocolate Chip Cookies

Pkg. (13 oz.) chocolate chips
1 c. shortening
Combine:
2½ c. flour
1 tsp. salt
1 tsp. soda
½ tsp. water
¾ c. white sugar
½ c. + 2 tbsp. brown sugar
2 eggs
Cream:
Shortening and sugars, then add eggs and water. Combine flour, salt and soda and add creamed mixture and stir in the melted chocolate chips and optional nuts. Bake at 375°F for 8-10 minutes.
From the kitchen of Catherine G.

Give God what's right – not what's left.

Man's way leads to a hopeless end – God's way leads to an endless hope.

A lot of kneeling will keep you in good standing.

He who kneels before God can stand before anyone.

Mother's Chocolate Chip Cookies

Chocolate chip cookies.

3/4 C brown sugar   1 C shortening
3/4 C white sugar   2 eggs
2 C flour   1 t soda
2 C chips   1/2 t water
1 C nuts 1 t vanilla   1 t salt
Beat shortening + sugars + vanilla, water, + eggs until light & fluffy, mix flour, salt soda. Blend into shortening mixture stir in chips + nuts. drop by spoon onto cookie sheet. Bake 8 min. at 350°

From the kitchen of Irene T.

60s Songs Changed

Some of the artists of the 60s are revising their hits, with new lyrics to accommodate aging baby boomers who can remember doing the 'Limbo' as if it were yesterday.

They include:

Bobby Darin --- Splish, Splash, I Was Havin' a Flash

Herman's Hermits --- Mrs. Brown, You've Got a Lovely Walker

Ringo Starr --- I Get By With a Little Help from Depends

The Bee Gees --- How Can You Mend A Broken Hip?

Roberta Flack--- The First Time Ever I Forgot Your Face

Johnny Nash --- I Can't See Clearly Now.

Cappuccino Chocolate Chip Cookies

2 tsp. instant coffee granules

1 tbsp. coffee flavored liqueur or milk

1 c. firmly packed brown sugar

1 c. Land of Lakes butter, softened

½ c. sugar

One oz. square semi-sweet baking chocolate, melted, cooled

2 eggs

1 tsp. vanilla

2½ c. all-purpose flour

1 tsp. baking soda

1 tsp. ground cinnamon

⅛ tsp. salt

12 oz. pkg. (2 c.) semi-sweet real chocolate chips

Drizzle:

3 oz. white baking bar

2 tsp. shortening

Heat oven to 375°F. Dissolve coffee granules in coffee liqueur or milk in a small bowl. Combine brown sugar, sugar and butter in large mixer bowl. Beat at medium speed, scraping bowl often, until well mixed. (1-2 minutes) Add coffee mixture, cooled melted chocolate, eggs and vanilla; continue beating until well mixed (1-2 minutes). Reduce speed to low; add flour, baking soda, cinnamon and salt. Beat until well mixed. Stir in chocolate chips by hand. Drop dough by rounded teaspoonful two inches apart onto ungreased cookie sheets. Bake at 375°F for 8-10 minutes or until golden brown. Cool completely. Melt white baking bar and shortening in 1-quart saucepan over low heat, stirring occasionally, until smooth (4-6 minutes). Drizzle over cooled cookies. Makes 5 dozen cookies. 110 calories per cookie!!!!!!! From the kitchen of Phyliss T.

Often when we lose hope and think this is the end, GOD smiles from above and says, "Relax, sweetheart, it's just a bend, not the end!"

When GOD solves your problems, you have faith in HIS abilities; when GOD doesn't solve your problems HE has faith in your abilities.

Chocolate Butter Sweets

½ c. butter or oleo
½ c. confectioners' sugar (powdered sugar)
¼ tsp. salt
1 tsp. vanilla
1 – 1¼ c. flour

Cream the butter. Add sugar, salt and vanilla. Cream well. Gradually add flour. Shape by teaspoonfuls into balls. Place on un-greased cookie sheet. Press hole in the center. Bake at 350° F. for 12 to 15 minutes. Fill while warm with filling.

Filling:

3 oz. cream cheese
1 c. confectioners' sugar
2 tbsp. flour
1 tsp. vanilla
½ c. chopped nuts
½ c. coconut

Soften cream cheese. Blend in sugar, flour and vanilla. Cream well. Add nuts and coconut. Fill holes of baked product.

Frosting:

½ c. chocolate chips
2 tbsp. butter
2 tbsp. water
½ c. confectioners' sugar

Melt the chips, butter, and water over a low heat. Add the confectioners' sugar. Beat until smooth. Frost cookies
From the kitchen of Willie Faye J.

Payday Bars

Crust:
1½ c. flour,
2/3 c. brown sugar
½ tsp. baking powder
½ c. margarine
2 egg yolks
1 tsp. vanilla
2 tsp. water
Mix flour, sugar, and baking powder, cut in margarine. Mix egg yolks, water and vanilla. Add to flour mixture and mix well. Pat out on jelly roll pan. Bake at <u>350°</u> <u>F</u>. for 12 minutes.

Topping:
¾ c. white Karo
1 pkg. peanut butter chips
Melt together in pan and pour over the baked sheet. Cut into 2 inch x 4 inch bars.
From the kitchen of Phyliss T.

Rocky Road Fudge Bars

Bar:
½ c. margarine or butter
½ to 1 c. chopped nuts
Square (1 oz.) unsweetened chocolate or 1 envelope pre-melted, unsweetened baking chocolate flavor
1 c. sugar &1 tsp. vanilla & 2 eggs
1 c. all purpose or unbleached flour
1 tsp. baking powder

Filling:
8 oz. pkg. cream cheese, softened (Reserve 2 oz. for frosting)
½ c. sugar
2 tsp. flour
¼ c. margarine or butter, softened
Egg
½ tsp. vanilla
¼ c. chopped nuts
6 oz. pkg. (1 c.) semi sweet chocolate chips if desired

Frosting:
2 c. miniature marsh mellows and
¼ c. margarine or butter
Square (1 oz.) unsweetened chocolate or 1 envelope pre-melted unsweetened baking chocolate flavor
2 oz. reserved cream cheese
¼ c. milk

3 c. powdered sugar

1 tsp. vanilla

Heat oven to 350° F. Grease (not oil) and flour 13-inch x 9-inch pan. In large saucepan over low heat, melt ½ cup margarine and 1 square chocolate (Lightly spoon flour into measuring cup; level off.) Add remaining Bar ingredients; mix well. Spread in prepared pan. In small bowl, combine 6 oz. cream cheese with next five Filling ingredients. Beat 1 minute at medium spread until smooth and fluffy; stir in nuts. Spread over chocolate mixture. Sprinkle with chocolate chips. Bake at 530° F for 25-35 minutes or until toothpick inserted in center comes out clean. Remove from oven; sprinkle with marsh mellows. Bake 2 minutes longer. In large saucepan, over low heat, melt ¼ cup margarine, 1 square chocolate, remaining 2 ounce. Cream cheese and milk. Stir in powdered sugar and vanilla until smooth. Immediately pour over marsh mellows and swirl together. Cool; cut into bars. Store in refrigerator. 3-4 dozen bars.

From the kitchen of Catherine G.

Elephant Ears

Mix Together:

1 pkg. dry yeast

¼ c. warm water (105-115° F.)

Sift Together:

2 c. flour

1½ tbsp. sugar

½ tsp. salt

Cut into flour mixture:

1 c. butter

Combine with yeast mixture:

½ c. scaled milk

Egg yolk

Stir all the above together:

Mix well. Chill dough 2 hours. Turn dough out onto floured surface, knead 2 minutes. Cover and let rest 10 minutes. Roll dough into18-inch x 10-inch rectangle on floured surface. Brush with melted butter.

Combine:

2 c. sugar

1 tbsp. and ½ tsp. cinnamon Sprinkle 1 cup of the sugar mixture over the dough. Roll up jelly roll fashion, starting at long side. Place seam side down. Using sewing thread, cut into 18 – 1 inch slices. Sprinkle some of the sugar mixture over wax paper. Roll each of the slices in sugar

mixture, turning once. Place on a cookie sheet.

Put on the slices:

¼ c. melted butter

½ c. chopped pecans

remaining cup sugar mixture

Bake at 400° F. for 10 minutes.

Cool on wire racks.

From the kitchen of Sue Ann T.

Oatmeal Cookies

¾ c. oleo (1½ sticks)

½ c. white sugar

½ c. brown sugar

1 egg

1 tsp. vanilla

¾ c. sifted flour

1½ c. oats

¼ tsp. baking soda & ½ tsp. salt

½ c. chopped pecans

Cream softened butter and sugar, continue beating – add egg and vanilla.   Sift dry ingredients together and gradually add to butter mixture. Chill. Roll in roll. Slice a inch thick. Place on cookie sheet. Bake at 350° F., 8-10 min.

From the kitchen of Sara H.

Oatmeal Cookies

Combine:

1 c. white sugar

½ tsp. salt

1 c. shortening

1 c. raisins, boiled in water with cover. Let cool

Add:

5 tbsp. raisin liquid

Add:

1 tsp. soda

2 eggs

2 c. flour

1 tsp. cinnamon

1 tsp. nutmeg

1 c. walnuts

1 tsp vanilla

Drop by spoonfuls on cookie sheets. Bake at 375° F. For 30-35 minutes.

From the kitchen of Ethel A.

Oatmeal Cookies

1¾ c. flour

6 tbsp. milk

¾ tsp. soda

2 c. oatmeal

1 c. raisins or nuts

1 tsp. cinnamon

½ tsp. cloves and ½ tsp. allspices

2 eggs

½ c. shortening
1 c. sugar and ½ tsp. salt
Place shortening in mixing bowl and cream.
Second, add 1 c. sugar to shortening and cream well.
Third, add 2 eggs and heat hard.
Fourth, measure 1¾ cup flour.
Fifth, measure 1 cup of raisins or nuts. And add 1 or 2 tablespoons of the flour. This keeps the raisins from sticking together. Stir.
Sixth, put the soda into the milk, stir well and add to egg, sugar and shortening mixture.
Seventh, add the flour next the oatmeal, cinnamon, salt, cloves, allspice, and floured raisins or nuts. More milk may be added if necessary. The batter should be so thick that it is necessary to scrap form end of spoon when dropping it.
Eight, drop by spoonfuls about the size of a small walnut on greased baking tins 1½ inches apart.
Ninth, bake in oven at 375° F. for 10 to 15 minutes.
4-H Demonstration Recipe from the kitchen of Melba R.

Pumpkin Bars

2½ c. sugar
4 med. Eggs, beaten
1 c. powdered milk
Large can pumpkin (29 oz.)
1 c. vegetable oil or (may have ½ c. oil and ½ c. applesauce)
1 tbsp. vanilla
5 tbsp. cinnamon (Yes, 5 tbsp)
5 c. flour (use part whole wheat)
1½ tsp. baking soda
2 tbsp. baking powder
1 – 2 tsp. salt
1½ c. raisins
1½ c. pecans or walnuts
Blend together sugar, eggs, powdered milk, pumpkin, oil and vanilla. Gently stir the cinnamon into the mixture. Stir in dry ingredients. Then add raisins and nuts. Divide the batter into two sheet cake pans. Bake for 15 minutes at 350° F. Cut into bars. (May drop by spoonfuls and make cookies if desired)
From the kitchen of Linda A.

"I believe that you should always leave loved ones with loving words. It may be the last time you see them.

Date Cookies

1 c. shortening
2 c. brown sugar
2 eggs
½ c. buttermilk
1 tsp. vanilla
3½ c. flour
1 tsp. salt
1 tsp. soda

Cream shortening, sugar and eggs. Stir in milk and vanilla. Add sifted flour, soda, and salt. Drop tablespoon size dough onto ungreased baking sheet. Place ½ tablespoon date filling on dough, cover with ½ tablespoon dough.

Bake 10 to 12 minutes at 400° F.

Date Filling:
Stir together:
2 c. dates, cut small
¾ c. sugar
¾ c. water.

Cook until thick stirring constantly
Add: ½ c. chopped nuts.
Cool. Makes 5 – 6 dozen.

From the kitchen of Willie Fay J.

Popcorn Balls

5 qt popped corn
2 c. sugar
1½ c. water
½ c. light corn syrup
1 tsp vinegar
1 tsp. vanilla
1/3 tsp. salt

Keep popcorn hot and crisp in a slow oven (300-325° F.) Cook sugar, water, salt, and corn syrup to very hard ball stage. Add vinegar and vanilla; cook to light crack stage. Slowly pour over popped corn; stir well to coat every kernel. Press in balls. Use fat on hands if necessary. Makes 20 popcorn balls.

From the kitchen of Catherine G.

Mrs. Field's Cookies

(Works well to cut in half)

2 c. butter, creamed
2 c. sugar
2 c. brown sugar
4 eggs
2 tsp. vanilla
5 c. oatmeal
4 c. flour
2 tsp. baking powder
1 tsp. salt
2 tsp. soda
24 oz. chocolate chips
18 oz. Hershey bar, grated

3 c. nuts, chopped

Mix together creamed butter, both sugars, eggs and vanilla. Put small amount of oatmeal at a time in blender and turn into powder. Stir in all the remaining ingredients. Put on a cookie sheet – golf ball size 2 inches apart. Bake at 375° F. for about 10 minutes. (For just Oatmeal cookies, add lots of raisins.) If smaller cookies desired, make one inch balls and bake for 6 minutes or more.

From the kitchen of Phyliss T.

Snickerdoodles

1½ c. soft shortening (part butter)
2¼ c. sugar
3 eggs
4 and 1/8 c. flour, sifted
3 tsp. cream of tartar
1½ tsp. soda
3/8 tsp. salt

Mix thoroughly shortening, sugar, and eggs. Sift together and stir in flour, cream of tartar, soda, and salt. Chill. Roll into balls the size of small walnuts.

Roll in mixture:

3 tbsp. sugar
3 tsp. cinnamon

Place 2 inches apart on ungreased baking sheet. Bake at 400° F. until lightly browned, but still soft for 8-10 minutes. Makes 7 dozen 2 inch cookies. These cookies puff up first, then flatten out.

From the kitchen of Linda A.

"Come work for the Lord. The work is hard, the hours are long and the pay is low. But the retirement benefits are out of this world."

Lemon Cookies

Cookies:
1 c. Crisco
1½ c. sugar
1 tbsp. lemon extract
2 eggs
2¼ c. flour
1 tsp. baking soda
2 tsp. cream of tartar
Mix well the Crisco, sugar, lemon extract and eggs. Mix flour, soda and cream of tartar. Add to creamed mixture. Make golf size balls, put on cookie sheet. Bake at 350° F. for 10 minutes. Cool and ice. Best taste the next day.

Icing:
Stick butter, softened
¼ c. lemon juice
1 lb. powdered sugar
Mix together and use as icing. Spread icing on each cookie.
Adapted from Cookie Basket
From the kitchen of Catherine G.

Don't count the years – count the memories…..

Little Bits

12 graham crackers
3 eggs, separated
¾ c. sugar
2 – 8 oz. cream cheese, softened
cream egg yolks, sugar and cream cheese until fluffy. Beat egg whites till stiff. Fold egg whites into creamed mixture. Butter insides of 2 muffin pans. Spoon crushed graham crackers in each muffin tin to coat inside of pans. Spoon cream mixture into muffin tins, filling them ¾ full. Bake at 350° F. for 20 minutes Cool 10-15 minutes. Centers will fall, forming indentations. Carefully remove from muffin tins. Spoon 1 teaspoon sour cream mixture into the indentations. Store in refrigerator. Yield is 4 dozen.

Sour Cream Filling:
1 – 8 oz. carton sour cream
¾ c. sugar
½ tsp. vanilla
Combine all ingredients in 9 inch pie plate. Stir well. Bake at 400° F. for 5 minutes. Stir well and bake for an additional 3 minutes. Yields 1 cup filling.
From the kitchen of Catherine G.

Pecan Puffs

Preheat oven to 300° F.

Beat until soft:

½ c. butter

Add and blend until creamy:

2 tbsp. sugar

Add:

1 tsp. vanilla

Grind in a nut grinder 1 c. pecan
    meats

Sift before measuring:

1 c. cake flour

Stir the pecans and the flour into
the butter mixture. Roll the
dough into small balls.   Place
balls on a greased baking sheet
and bake for about 20 minutes.
Roll while still hot in
Confectioners' sugar.   To glaze,
put the sheet back into the oven
for a minute. Cool and serve.
Rich and devastating.

From the kitchen of Catherine G

Sugar Cookies

2 sticks of oleo or butter (1 c.)

1 c. sugar

2 large eggs

1 tsp. vanilla

3¾ c. all-purpose flour

2 tsp. baking powder

¼ c. heavy cream

Beat butter and sugar until fluffy.
Add eggs and vanilla. Use low
speed. Add flour, baking powder
and cream until blended. Divide
dough in half and wrap in saran
wrap and then chill for 3 hours.
Roll dough to ½ inch thick rolls
and cut with cookie cutters. Bake
at 350° F. for 12 minutes.

From the kitchen of Alecia M.

Melt In Your Mouth Sugar Cookie

1 c. butter

1 c. powdered sugar

1 c. white sugar

1 c. vegetable oil

2 eggs

1 tsp. vanilla

1 tsp. cream of tartar

4¼ c. flour

1 tsp. baking soda

1 tsp. salt

Preheat oven to 350° F. Cream
butter and sugars, then mix in oil
and eggs. Add vanilla, and cream
of tartar. Mix dry ingredients and
add to creamed mixture. Form
into 1 inch balls and roll in sugar.
Place on cookie sheet (ungreased)
and flatten with hand. Bake 10-12
minutes.

Unknown kitchen

Mother's Sugar Cookie

¾ c. and 1½ tbsp. butter
2 eggs
1½ c. sugar
1 tsp. vanilla
3 c. flour
1 tsp. soda
¼ tsp. salt
Mix and roll into balls, place on cookie sheet and mash with a glass dipped in sugar. Bake at 350° F. for 10-12 minutes.
From the kitchen of Irene T.

Sugar Cookie Icing

1 c. shortening
Pound powdered sugar
¼ c. milk
1 pinch salt
1 tsp. flavoring (vanilla or almond extract)
Cream shortening, powdered sugar
Add milk (adding alternately)
Add salt and flavoring.
Beat mixture for about 5 minutes until fluffy.
From the kitchen of Alecia M.

Norma's Cheese Straws

½ lb. butter
½ lb. sharp cheese
2 c. flour
2 c. rice crisp
No salt
Mix ingredients and roll into small balls size. Place on un-greased cookie sheet and flatten with fork. Bake at 350 °F. for 10-15 minutes, until light brown.
From the kitchen of Norma C.

Old Fashion Molasses Cookies

1 c. sugar
1 c. shortening
1 c. sorghum
2 eggs, beaten
1 c. hot water or coffee
2 tsp. soda
¼ tsp. salt
1 tsp. ginger
9 c. flour
Cream shortening and sugar.
Add other ingredients in order given and work to soft dough.
Roll to about ¼ inch thickness

or (slightly thicker) cut in desired shapes and bake in moderate oven until done.

From the kitchen of Ethel A.

No Baked Cookies

2 c. sugar

6 tbsp. cola

Stick of butter

½ c. milk

Combine and bring to a boil for 3 minutes. Take off the heat and add:

2 c. quick oats

1 tsp. vanilla

Stir, then drop on wax paper. Let cool down before serving

From the kitchen of Susan M.

Praline-Topped Brown Sugar Slices

1 c. brown sugar, firmly packed

1 c. butter, softened

1 egg

2 tbsp. half & half

1½ tsp. vanilla

3 c. all-purpose flour

½ tsp. baking powder

¼ tsp. baking soda

¼ tsp. salt

2/3 c. pecans, finely chopped

Combine brown sugar and butter in large bowl. Beat at medium speed, scraping bowl often, until creamy. Add egg, half and half and vanilla; continue beating until well mixed. Reduce speed to low; add flour, baking powder, baking soda and salt. Beat until well mixed. Stir in chopped pecans by hand. Divide dough in half; shape each half into 8½-inch long roll. Wrap each roll in plastic food wrap. Refrigerate until firm (1 to 2 hours.). Heat oven to 375° F. Cut rolls into ¼-inch slices with sharp knife. Place 1 inch apart on ungreased cookie sheets. Bake for 7 to 9 minutes. Or until edges are lightly browned.   Remove from cookie sheets. Cool cookies completely on cooling racks over waxed paper. Makes 5½ dozen.

Topping:

1 c. brown sugar, firmly packed

¼ c. butter

¼ c. half & half

1¼ c. powdered sugar

½ c. pecans, finely chopped, toasted

Combine brown sugar, butter and half and half in 3-quart saucepan. Cook over medium-high heat, stirring occasionally, until mixture comes to a full boil (3 to 4 minutes). Reduce heat to

medium-low. Continue cooking, without stirring, for 1 minute. Remove saucepan from heat. Stir in powdered sugar and chopped pecans. Let stand until desired spreading consistency (1 to 2 minutes). Quickly spread over cooled cookies. If the praline topping hardens too quickly, stir in a few drops of hot water. Adapted from the recipe of the same title from Land O'Lakes Recipe page.
From the kitchen of Phyliss T.

"If you're headed in the wrong direction, God allows U-turns."

Pecan Sugar Free Cookies

1¼ c. whole wheat flour
1 tsp. baking powder
¼ tsp. baking soda
¼ tsp. salt
½ c. butter or margarine
3 tbsp. brown sugar replacement (e.g. Sugar Twin)
9 tbsp. SPLENDA® Granular
1 egg, lightly beaten
½ tsp. vanilla extract

1½ c. chopped pecans
Preheat the oven to 375 °F. Sift together flour, baking powder, baking soda, and salt. In a mixing bowl, cream together butter and sugar replacements. Beat in egg and vanilla. Mix in flour mixture. Stir in pecans. Drop by rounded teaspoon onto ungreased baking sheet. Bake in preheated oven for about 10 minutes. Cool cookies slightly before removing from pan. Yields 2 dozen.

Blondies

2 sticks butter
Box light brown sugar
2 eggs
2 c. flour
2 tsp. flour
2 tsp. baking powder
Preheat oven to 350° F. Melt butter, add eggs, brown sugar and vanilla. Mix well, add flour and baking powder. Mix well. Add whatever you like – chocolate chips – nuts – coconut, etc. Pour into 9-inch x 13-inch pan. Bake 20-25 minutes or until light brown and edges pull away from pan.
From the kitchen Teresa M.

Cream Cheese Christmas Bars

1 can crescent rolls, unrolled in a 19 inch crescent pan
2 - 8 oz. cream cheese
1 c. sugar
2 tsp. vanilla
mix and spread on crescent rolls:
Can crescent rolls, unrolled and
    lay over it
Stick butter, melted
Add:
1 c. sugar
2 tsp. cinnamon
Pour over second layer.   Bake at 350°F. for 30-40 minutes. Cool and cut in small squares.
From the kitchen of Paula H.

Oatmeal Toffee Cookies

1 c. (2 sticks) butter or margarine
2 eggs
2 c. light brown sugar
2 tsp. vanilla
1¾ c. flour
1 tsp. baking soda
1 tsp. cinnamon
½ tsp. salt
3 c. quick cooking oats
10 oz. Pkg. Heath Bits' O Brickle Almond Toffee Bits
1 c. sweetened coconut (optional)
Heat oven to 375° F. Use lightly greased cookie sheets.   Beat butter, eggs, brown sugar and vanilla in a large bowl until well blended.   Add flour, baking soda, cinnamon and salt; beat until well blended. Stir in oats, toffee bits and coconut, if desired with spoon. Drop dough by rounded teaspoon about 2 inches apart onto cookie sheet and bake for 10-12 minutes.
From the kitchen of Debbie W.

Cool Whip Cookies

Pkg. cake mix (any flavor)
4½ oz. Cool Whip or 2 c.
1 egg
½ c. powdered sugar
1 tsp. vanilla
Combine cake mix, cool whip, egg and vanilla, mixing well. Drop by teaspoon into powdered sugar until cooled.
From the kitchen of Pat J.

Buttery Toffee Cookies

From the kitchen of Debbie W.

1 c. butter, softened
1 c. sugar
2 eggs and 1 tsp. vanilla
2 ½ c. flour
1 tsp. baking soda
½ tsp. salt
8 oz. pkg. milk chocolate toffee
   bits

Heat oven to 350° F. Combine butter, sugar, eggs and vanilla in large mixer bowl. Beat at medium speed, scraping bowl, until creamy. Reduce Speed to low; add flour, baking soda and salt. Beat until well mixed. Stir in toffee bits by hand. Drop dough by rounded teaspoonfuls onto ungreased cookie sheets. Bake for 10 to 12 minutes or until lightly browned. let cool on cookie sheet for about 1 minutes then remove. Makes 4 dozen cookies.

Quit Worrying

Life has dealt you a blow and all you do is sit and worry. Have you forgotten that I am here to take all your burdens and carry them for you? Or do you just enjoy fretting over every little thing that comes your way?
Author unknown.

Chapter 11
Cakes and Icings

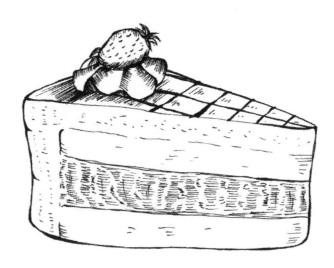

Index of Cakes and Icing Recipes

Angel Food Cake

11 egg whites
1 tsp. cream of tartar
1½ c. sugar and 1 tsp. vanilla
1 c. flour or cake flour
Beat the whites, add salt, cream of tartar and vanilla, and beat again, until it stands in stiff peaks. Fold in the sugar and then the flour that has been sifted five times. Pour it into a dry angel food cake pan. Bake in moderate oven at 350° F. for 45 minutes.
From the kitchen of Irene T.

Angel Food Cake

1½ c. egg whites
1½ tsp. cream of tartar
1 c. sugar and ⅛ tsp. salt
1 tsp. vanilla
1 c. cake flour
1½ c. confectioners' sugar
Beat egg whites until feathery; add cream of tartar. Beat until stiff, but not dry. Add sugar, little at a time. Add salt and vanilla. Sift the cake flour and confectionary sugar and sift three times. Then sift into mixture and fold in. Bake in tube pan for 1 hour and 5 minutes at 325° F.
From the kitchen of Ethel A.

Blackberry Snack Cake

¾ c. flour
¾ c. sugar
1½ tsp. baking powder
Dash of salt
Add ½ c. milk
Mix ingredients, put in a pan
Add 2 cup blackberries layered on top.
2 tablespoon brown sugar sprinkled on top.
½ cup margarine, melted to pour over cake
Bake in 325° F. oven, 35 to 40 minutes.
From the kitchen of Phyllis T.

Mother's Prune Cake

1 c. margarine
1½ c. sugar
4½ eggs, beaten
4½ tbsp. sour cream
3 c. flour
¾ tsp. salt
1½ tsp. allspice
3 tsp. cinnamon (optional)
1½ tsp. soda
1½ tsp. vanilla
1½ c. prunes cut up with shears
Cream butter and sugar and stir in the eggs and sour cream. Add

sifted flour, salt, allspice, and cinnamon. Dissolve soda in small amount of hot water and add to mixture. Add vanilla and prunes. Pour into two - 9 inch cake pans, which have been oiled and dusted with flour. Bake in oven at 350° F. for 25-35 minutes or until done.

Filling:
3 eggs
1½ c. sugar,
1½ c. chopped prunes
Beat well and cook until thick.
Cover cake when filling has cooked.
From the kitchen of Irene T.

Prune Cake

Combine dry ingredients
2 c. flour
2 c. sugar
2 tsp. soda
1 tsp. cloves
2 tsp. cinnamon
1 tsp. nutmeg
1 tsp. allspice
1 c. prunes, chopped
1 c. buttermilk
1 c. corn oil
3 each eggs. beaten
(sometimes I add a tsp. vanilla)
Combine all ingredients. Bake at 350° F. for 1½ hours in a bunt pan.

Frosting

Cream and Ice Cake:
¼ c. butter
¾ c. buttermilk
1½ tsp. dark corn syrup
1½ c. sugar
2 tsp. vanilla extract
Cream together and ice the cake.

Aunt Eula's Strawberry Cake

White cake mix (Betty Crocker)
Pkg. strawberry jello
½ c. Wesson oil
½ c. crushed strawberries
½ c. water
4 eggs
Combine cake mix and jello
Add Wesson oil, strawberries, and water and beat 2 minutes. Beat the eggs separately and add to mixture
Beat 2 more minutes. Makes 2 layers. Bake at 350° F. for 30 minutes.

Icing: Mix until creamy
Stick margarine,
Pound package powdered sugar
½ cup strawberries.
From the kitchen of Eula J.

Strawberry Icebox Cake

Cut a small angel food cake into cubes and place in triffle bowl.

1 (3 oz.) pkg. instant vanilla pudding

1 c. cold dry milk

1 pt. vanilla ice cream

Beat together pudding, milk and ice cream until smooth. Pour over cake

Make topping.

1 small package strawberry jello dissolve in 1 cup boiling water.

Stir into this 1 large package frozen strawberries until they fall apart.

Cool until it is jelly-like consistency. Pour over cake. Refrigerate until jello sets. Serve immediately.

From the kitchen of Linda A.

Strawberry Cream Cake with Icing

1½ c. sugar

½ c. margarine

3 eggs, separated

1 c. milk

2 c. flour

2 tsp. baking powder

1 tsp. vanilla

2 sliced fresh strawberries

Cream sugar and margarine. Add egg yolks and cream again. Add flour and baking powder alternately with milk. Fold in egg whites that have been beaten stiff. Add vanilla. Bake 30-35 minutes at 350° F. in a 13-inch x 9-inch pan.

Icing:

5 tbsp. flour and 1 c. milk

1 c. sugar

1 tsp. vanilla

1 c. margarine

[double batch, at least]

Cook flour and milk together until thick. Stir constantly. Set aside to cool; this must be cold before you mix in the next ingredients. Cream sugar, margarine and vanilla with mixer until light in color and creamy. Add flour and milk mixture. Beat until spreading consistency like whipped cream. Slice cake in half and then each square in half to make 4 layers. Using 3 layers for strawberry cake – between each layer, put icing, strawberries and icing, and on top complete with icing, strawberries and icing.

From the kitchen of Flora F.

Pressed Fruit Cake

1 lb. dried apricots
1 lb. dried apples
1 lb. seedless raisins
1 lb. pitted prunes
1 lb. dried peaches
1 lb. pitted dates
1 lb. dried figs
1 lb. dried walnuts
1 lb. pecans
1 fresh orange with peel (seeds
    removed)
1 c. granulated sugar

Put though food grinder all the fruits and nuts. Add 1 tablespoon sugar from cup to each batch Then add the rest of the sugar, mixing thoroughly Pack firmly in two 9 inch x 5 inch loaf pans Place a heavy weight on top and leave overnight. Remove weight. Cover with plastic wrap and store in dark cool place 4 - 6 weeks. Remove from the pans. Makes up to 6 dozen slices.

From the kitchen of Phyllis T.

Pear Cake

2 c. sugar
¾ c. oil
3 eggs
2 tsp. vanilla
2 c. flour
2 tsp. cinnamon
1 tsp. soda
½ tsp. salt
3 c. chopped pears
1 c. pecan pieces

Cream sugar, oil, and eggs. Add vanilla. Mix in dry ingredients. Add pears and pecans. Bake in greased bundt or angel food pan at 350° F. for 1 hour.

From the kitchen of Earline G.

One-liners

Don't put a question mark where God puts a period.

Are you wrinkled with burden? Come to the church for a face-lift.

When praying, don't give God instructions - just report for duty.
Author Unknown

Lady Cake Italian Cream

1 box Duncan Hines Yellow cake
    mix
1 box coconut cream instant
    pudding
1½ c. coconut
1 c. nuts
4 eggs
1 c. water
¼ c. oil

Mix cake mix with eggs, water, oil and pudding. Add nuts. Bake according to box directions.
Ice with:
8 oz. cream cheese
1 lb. box powdered sugar
1½ stick margarine
1 tsp. vanilla.
Beat until smooth. Ice cake.
Toast 1½ cup coconut in 2 tablespoon of butter and sprinkle over the top of cake or add nuts to above icing.
From the kitchen of Phyliss T.

Grandma Todd's Banana Nut Cake

	Large	Medium	Small
Beat together:			
Butter	1 c.	1 c.	2/3 c.
Sugar	2½ c.	1⅞ c.	1¼ c.
Eggs	4	3	2
Add bananas to mixture:			
Mashed bananas	2 c.	1½ c.	1 c.
Combine and set aside:			
Buttermilk	½ c.	6 tbsp.	¼ c.
Soda	2 tsp.	1½ tsp.	1 tsp.

Combine dry ingredients and add to creamed mixture, alternating with buttermilk and soda:

	Large	Medium	Small
Salt	1 tsp.	¾ tsp.	½ tsp.
Flour	3 c.	2¼ c.	1½ c.
Cinnamon	1 tsp.	¾ tsp.	½ tsp.
Ground cloves	1 tsp.	¾ tsp.	½ tsp.

Then stir in the nuts and vanilla:

	Large	Medium	Small
pecans or walnuts (chopped or ground)	2 c.	1½ c.	1 c.
vanilla	2 tsp.	1½ tsp.	1 tsp.

Bake in an oiled and floured bunt cake pan for about one hour at 350° F. Cool. Ice with caramel icing.
From the kitchen of Lula Belle T.

Banana Nut Cake

½ c. butter or Crisco

1½ c. sugar

2 large eggs, lightly beaten

2 c. all purpose flour

½ tsp. salt

¾ tsp. soda

¼ c. of sour milk

1 c. bananas, mashed

1 c. chopped nuts

Blend together butter, sugar, eggs and bananas. Mix the soda and milk. Then alternate, mixing the flour/salt and the milk/soda to a creamed mix. Stir in nuts. Pour into a bundt pan. Bake at 350° F. for 30 minutes or until done.

From the kitchen of Mrs. Wells, Larry G's. grandmother.

Funnel Cake

2 eggs, beaten

1½ c. milk

2 c. flour

1 tsp. baking powder

½ tsp. cinnamon

½ tsp. salt

¼ c. sugar

Mix ingredients and beat real smooth. Heat it with 2 cup oil to 360° F. Fry until brown. Remove and drain on paper towels. Sift powdered sugar on top and serve.

From the kitchen of Earline G.

Pumpkin Pound Cake

3 c. sugar

3 eggs and 1 c. oil

2 c. (or one can) pumpkin

3 c. flour and ½ tsp. soda

2 tsp. baking powder

1 tsp. salt

2 tsp. cinnamon

1 tsp. nutmeg

1 tsp. allspice

Mix sugar, eggs and oil in a bowl. Add pumpkin. Mix well. Measure flour and other dry ingredients, sift twice, then add to first mixture. Bake in tube pan that has been greased and floured. Bake 35 minutes. at 350° F, then reduce heat to 275° F. and bake for 30 minutes. Keeps moist for days.

From the kitchen of Darlene P.

Actual Church Signs

 "CHURCH PARKING - FOR MEMBERS ONLY!" Trespassers will be baptized!

"Free Trip to Heaven. Details Inside!"

"Try our Sundays. They are better than Baskin-Robbins."

An ad for one Church has a picture of two hands holding stone tablets on which the Ten Commandments are inscribed and a headline that reads, - "For Fast Relief, Take Two Tablets.

Apple Cake

Preparing the Cake:

1 c. oil

2 c. sugar

2 eggs

1 tsp. vanilla

1 tsp. salt

1 tsp. baking soda

2 tsp. baking powder

2 ½ c. flour

3 c. apples, chopped

Beat oil, sugar, eggs, and vanilla together. Blend in dry ingredients. Stir in apples. Spread into lightly oiled 13 inch x 9 inch pan.

Topping:

1/3 c. brown sugar

1 tsp. cinnamon

½ c. chopped nuts (1 use pecan pieces, they are much smaller.)

Combine and sprinkle over cake.

Bake at 350° F. for 40 minutes.

Remove from the oven. Serve warm with vanilla sauce poured over entire cake.

Vanilla Sauce:

½ c. butter

1½ c. whipping cream

1 c. sugar

2 tbsp. flour

2 tsp. vanilla

Combine all ingredients except vanilla. Cook in saucepan over medium heat, stirring often, until thickened. Add vanilla and stir. Pour over cake and serve.

From the kitchen of Sonya C.

Robbie's Killer Apple Cake

4 c. apples, peeled sliced
2 c. sugar
2 c. flour
1½ tsp. baking soda
2 tsp. cinnamon and 1 tsp. salt
2 each eggs
¾ c. vegetable oil
2 tsp. vanilla extract
1 c. pecans chopped

Preheat oven to 350° F.

In large bowl mix apples and sugar. Add all dry ingredients. In 2nd bowl beat eggs, oil and vanilla. Stir egg mixture into apples. Blend until fully moist. Stir in pecans and pour into 13-inch x 9-inch pan. Bake for 50 minutes.

Frosting (if you like a light frosting use this, I double it to cover the whole cake)

1 c. sugar
½ c. butter
½ c. evaporated milk or heavy
    cream
1 tsp. vanilla extract

Heat all ingredients to boiling. Pour over warm cake from oven. Wait for a little while before serving.
From the kitchen of Robbie W.

Fresh Apple Cake

1½ c. cooking oil
2 c. sugar
3 c. flour
1 tsp. soda
2 tsp. vanilla
2 eggs
1 tsp. salt
1 c. nuts
3 c. fresh apples, chopped

Mix all ingredients well, then add apples last. You may wish to add raisins if desired. Bake at 350° F. for 50 minutes. (Sift powdered sugar on top after coming out of the oven.)
From the kitchen of Melba R.

German Chocolate Cake

1 pkg. German chocolate
2 c. sugar
1 c. margarine
2½ c. flour
4 egg yolks, beaten
1 c. buttermilk

1 tsp. soda

1 tsp. vanilla

¼ tsp. salt

4 egg whites

Hersey's Plain Chocolate Bar

¼ c. boiling water

Cream the sugar and butter. Add well beaten egg yolks. Add ¾ cup of the buttermilk. Sift flour and salt. Add soda to the remaining buttermilk and add. Melt chocolate in the boiling water and add. Add vanilla and stiffly beaten egg whites. Bake it at 350° F. for 25 minutes. Use German Chocolate Icing. From the kitchen of Catherine G.

Chocolate Sheet Cake

Preheat oven to 400° F.

2 c. flour

2 c. sugar

1 c. water

1 stick margarine

½ c. Crisco

6 tbsp. cocoa

1 tbsp. vanilla

2 eggs

½ c. buttermilk

1 tsp. baking soda

Sift together flour and sugar. In a separate bowl, mix water, margarine, Crisco, and cocoa. Put on stove top and bring to a boil, stirring constantly. Add in the flour and sugar mix. Mix well. Add in the vanilla, eggs, butter milk, and baking soda. Mix well and pour into greased sheet cake pan and bake for 30 minutes at 350° F. Adding 1 cup nuts optional.

Frosting:

1 stick margarine

4 tbsp. cocoa

1 box powdered sugar

1 tsp. vanilla

1 c. nuts

Mix oleo and cocoa. Bring to a boil, stirring constantly. Remove from heat. Add powdered sugar, vanilla and nuts. Mix well and spread on cake while hot.

From the kitchen of Paula H.

Chocolate Cake and Icing

Cake:

1 lb. brown sugar – light
2 c. sifted flour
3 squares chocolate
1 c. hot water
¼ lb. margarine
½ c. sour milk
1¼ tsp. baking soda
2 eggs
1 tsp. vanilla

Mix together brown sugar and flour. Melt chocolate, hot water and margarine in saucepan. Add this to flour mixture, blend well. Combine sour milk and baking soda. Mix well and then add eggs and vanilla. Thoroughly blend. Bake in a greased 13 inch x 9 inch pan for 30 - 40 minutes at 375° F.

Icing:

1½ squares chocolate
1 c. granulated sugar
1 tsp. vanilla
3 tbsp. cornstarch
1 c. boiling water
1 tbsp. margarine
Icing:
Melt chocolate; add cornstarch,

sugar and boiling water. Boil until thick, stirring constantly, and then add vanilla and margarine. Put on cool cake while icing is still hot. From the kitchen of Flora F.

Chocolate Sheet Cake

2 c. flour
2 c. sugar
½ tsp. salt
1 c. water
½ c. shortening
2 tbsp. cocoa
1 stick margarine
2 eggs
1 tsp. soda
½ c. buttermilk
1 tsp. vanilla

Combine the flour, sugar and salt. Boil the water, shortening, cocoa and margarine. Pour over the dry ingredients. Add eggs, one at a time, beating well after each. Add soda to buttermilk and add to mixture. Add vanilla. Pour into greased and floured sheet cake pan and bake for 20 minutes at 350° F.

Frosting:

1 stick margarine and 6 tbsp. milk

3 tbsp. cocoa and1 tsp. vanilla

1 box powdered sugar

½ c. nuts

Bring to a boil the margarine, milk, and cocoa. Beat in the powdered sugar and vanilla. Add nuts.

From the kitchen of Bobbye P. Melinda A. and Aukse H.

Chocolate Cake

Cream:

Stick margarine

½ c. shortening

4 tbsp. cocoa

1 c. water

Boil the above until melted. Place in a mixing bowl and beat in sugar and vanilla.

Add:

2 c. sugar

1 tsp. vanilla

Combine and add:

2 c. flour

½ c. buttermilk

1 tsp. soda

2 tsp. cinnamon

Dash salt

Bake at 400° F. (10 minute-cupcakes or 20 minute-sheet cake.)

Icing:

1 stick margarine,

4 tsp. cocoa

6 tsp. milk

Mix and add 1 lb. powdered sugar and 1 tsp. vanilla and beat until smooth.

From the kitchen of Linda A.

Chocolate Trifle

Duncan Hines Devil's Food Cake (baked)

2 small boxes chocolate pudding (instant)

6 Kor candy bars (frozen) crumbled

1 c. pecans, chopped

Large Cool Whip

1/3 c. Khalua (Mexican coffee liquore)

Bake cake according to box instructions in a 9-inch x 13-inch pan. Then sprinkle Khalua over the cake while hot. Cool. Cut in squares. Make pudding. Chop the nuts and candy. In a large triffle or other glass bowl. Layer: cake, pudding, cool whip, nuts and candy. Then repeat layers ending with nuts and candy. Cool. Mother wanted the recipe but Cousin Mac never gave out her the recipe and now you know why!).

From the kitchen of Maurice M.

Ice Cream Candy Cane Cake

Angel food cake - slice horizontally into 3 layers

Extra creamy cool whip

¾ c. crushed peppermint candy

¼ c. coarsely, crushed peppermint candy

¼ c. water

Vanilla ice cream

Mix ¾ c. crushed candies with ¼ cup water to make a syrup.   On each layer of cake, spread 2 table spoon of syrup and ½ cup of cool whip topping.   Cover entire cake with remaining cool whip. Scoop vanilla ice cream around top of cake and sprinkle with ¼ cup coarsely, crushed candy. Freeze until ready to serve.

From the kitchen of Alecia M.

Never let an opportunity pass to say a kind and encouraging word to or about somebody. Praise good work, regardless of who did it.

Carrot Cake

2 c. all purpose flour (Consider substituting 1 c. whole wheat flour or 1 c. all purpose flour.)

2 c. granulated sugar (or use part Splenda)

2 tsp. baking soda

2 tsp. ground cinnamon

1 c. canola, or 1 c. olive oil

Unsweetened applesauce

3 eggs, beaten lightly

2 tsp. vanilla

1 1/3 c. cooked carrots, pureed

1 c. coconut

1 c. walnuts, optional

¾ c. crushed pineapple, drained

1 c. powdered milk

½ c. applesauce, optional

Preheat oven to 350° F.   Grease bundt cake pan. Sift dry ingredients in large bowl. In a mixer bowl, add oil, eggs, vanilla, powdered milk, and applesauce. Beat well. Gradually beat in dry ingredients. Fold in carrots, coconut, pineapple and nuts. Pour batter into pan, bake 1 hour till cake pulls from the pan edges. Cool for 10 minutes and un-mold. Cool to touch and ice with favorite creme cheese frosting.

From the kitchen of Nannette S.

Aunt Eula's Jello Cake

4 eggs
1 pkg. yellow cake mix
1 pkg. lemon jello
1/3 c. vegetable oil
¾ c. water

Mix the ingredients and pour into a 9 inch x 13 inch pan. Bake at 350° F. for 30 minutes. After taking from the oven, prick with a large fork.

Topping:
Juice from 1 orange
Juice from 1 lemon
2 c. powdered sugar

Mix topping ingredients and pour over the cake while the cake is still warm.

From the kitchen of Eula J.

Lemon Fluff

Pkg. lemon jello
1 c. sugar
1½ hot water
Can of Milnot, chilled and whipped
Can pineapple, crushed
Juice of lemon and grated rind, chilled
Juice of drained pineapple
Vanilla wafers

Combine jello, sugar, hot water, and juice of lemon and whip it. Mix in Milnot and pineapple juice. Pour into Pyrex pan lined with vanilla wafers. Add crumbs of vanilla wafers on top. Refrigerate until set up and then serve.

From the kitchen of Irene T.

Lemon Blossoms

18½ oz. pkg. yellow cake mix and
3½ oz. pkg. instant lemon pudding mix
4 large eggs
¾ c. vegetable oil

Preheat the oven to 350° F. Spray miniature muffin tins with vegetable oil cooking spray. Combine the cake mix, pudding mix, eggs and oil and blend well with an electric mixer until smooth, about 2 minutes. Pour a small amount of batter, filling each muffin tin half way. Bake for 12 minutes. Turn out onto a tea towel.

Glaze:
4 c. confectioners' sugar
1 c. fresh lemon juice
1 c. lemon, zested
3 tbsp. vegetable oil
3 tbsp. water

Sift the sugar into a mixing bowl. Add the lemon juice, zest, oil, and water. Mix with a spoon until smooth. With fingers, dip the cupcakes into the glaze while they're still warm, covering as much of the cake as possible, or spoon the glaze over the warm cupcakes, turning them to completely coat. Place on wire racks with waxed paper underneath to catch any drips. Let the glaze set thoroughly, about 1 hour, before storing in containers with tight-fitting lids. Ideal recipe for teas.

From Paula Dean's Home Cooking Show - Supper Club from the kitchen of Linda A.

A-P Cake and Funny Cake are both Pennsylvania Dutch recipes

A-P Cake

4 c. flour
2 heaping tsp. baking powder
2 c. brown sugar
¾ c. shortening
1 egg, beaten, and fill cup with milk
Sift flour and baking powder together. Add sugar and shortening; mix with pastry blender. Add the egg and milk, knead and bake at 350° F. for about 45 minutes in 2 greased pie tins.

From the kitchen of Patsy S.

Funny Cake

For two 9-inch funny cakes
Top Part:
1½ c. sugar
½ c. margarine
2 eggs
1 tsp. vanilla
2 c. flour
2 tsp. baking power
1 c. milk
Cream sugar, margarine and add eggs and vanilla and beat. Sift flour and baking powder. Add dry ingredients and milk alternately with egg mixture.

Lower Part:
½ c. cocoa
1 c. sugar
1 c. hot water
1 tsp. vanilla
Mix these ingredients and boil gently 1–2 minutes. Add vanilla and let cool before putting in two 9-inch pie pans. Top with ½ of batter in each 9 inch pan, dropping it on in large spoonfuls. Bake at 350° F for 35-40 minutes.

From the kitchen of Patsy S.

Blueberry Breakfast Cake

1 c. shortening
1½ c. sugar
2 tsp. vanilla
4 eggs, separated
1 tsp. baking soda
3 c. sifted flour
½ tsp. salt
2 tsp. baking powder
2/3 c. milk
½ c. sugar
3 c. blueberries
1 tbsp. flour
Confectioners' sugar

Cream shortening and sugar together. Add vanilla and egg yolks. Beat until light and fluffy. Sift together flour, baking powder and salt. Add alternately to cream mixture with milk. Beat egg whites until stiff - gradually add sugar and fold into batter. Add blueberries mixed with tablespoon flour. Pour into greased 9-inch x 9-inch x 2-inch pan. Bake in 350°F. degrees for 30-35 minutes or until cake tests done. When cool, sprinkle with confectioners' sugar.

From the kitchen of June T.

Aunt Flora's Black Walnut Cake

Cream:
1 c. butter or margarine
2 c. sugar
4 eggs
1 tsp. vanilla

Combine dry ingredients. Add to creamed mixture alternating with milk.

4 c. flour (save 2 tsp. for later)
4 tsp. baking power
½ tsp. salt
1¼ c. milk
1 c. black walnut meats, chopped and floured (take 2 tsp. from 4 c. of flour

Add nuts and pour into 2- 9 inch cake pans and bake at 350-375° F. for 35 minutes until done, test with a toothpick.

From the kitchen of Flora F.

Lazy Daisy Cake

12/3 c. flour
13/4 tsp. baking powder
1 c. sugar
¼ tsp. salt
1/3 c. shortening, softened
2/3 c. milk (not cold)
1 egg
1 tsp. flavoring
Sift dry ingredients together. Measure shortening in cup with milk. Add together with egg and flavoring. Beat well for 2 minutes. Bake in a 7 x 11 inch pan for 35 to 40 minutes at 350° F.

Icing:

Mix
3 tbsp. melted butter
5 tbsp. brown sugar
3 tbsp. cream
½ c. coconut.
Spread on warm cake. Place under broiler until mixture bubbles and browns, about 3 minutes.
From the kitchen of Pat J.

Talk To Me

I want you to forget a lot of things. Forget what was making you crazy. Forget the worry and the fretting because you know I'm in control.

But there's one thing I pray you never forget.
Please, don't forget to talk to Me - OFTEN! I love YOU! I want to hear your voice. I want you to include Me in on the things going on in your life. I want to hear you talk about your friends and family. Prayer is simply you having a conversation with Me. I want to be your dearest friend.
Author unknown

I Believe

I Believe... That just because two people argue, doesn't mean they don't love each other. And just because they don't argue, doesn't mean they <u>do</u> love each other.
I Believe... That no matter how good a friend is, they're going to hurt you every once in a while and you must forgive them for that.
I Believe... That true friendship continues to grow, even over the longest distance. Same goes for true love. **I Believe**... That you can do something in an instant that will give you heartache for life.

Kitty Litter Cake

Box spice or German chocolate
  cake mix
Box of white cake mix
Pkg. white sandwich cookies
1 lg. package vanilla instant pudding
  mix
A few drops green food coloring
12 small Tootsie Rolls or equivalent
Serving 'Dishes and Utensils'
NEW cat-litter box
NEW cat-litter box liner
NEW pooper scooper
Prepare and bake cake mixes,
according to directions, in any size
pan. Prepare pudding and chill.
Crumble cookies in small batches in
blender or food processor. Add a
few drops of green food coloring to
1 cup of cookie crumbs. Mix with a
fork or shake in a jar. Set aside.
2) When cakes are at room
temperature, crumble them into a
large bowl.
Toss with half of the remaining
cookie crumbs and enough pudding
to make the mixture moist but not
soggy.
Place liner in litter box and pour in
mixture.
3) Unwrap 3 Tootsie Rolls and heat
in a microwave until soft and
pliable.

Shape the blunt ends into slightly
curved points. Repeat with three
more rolls.
Bury the rolls decoratively in the
cake mixture. Sprinkle remaining
white cookie crumbs over the
mixture, then scatter green crumbs
lightly over top.
4) Heat 5 more Tootsie Rolls until
almost melted. Scrape them on top
of the cake and sprinkle with
crumbs from the 'litter box'.
Heat the remaining Tootsie Roll
until pliable and hang it over the
edge of the box.
Place box on a sheet of newspaper
and serve with new clean scooper.
Enjoy! 'Kitty **Litter** Cake' is
Great!!
From the kitchen of Linda A.

Be interested in others: their
pursuits, their work, their homes
and families.   Make merry with
those who rejoice; with those who
weep, mourn. Let everyone you
meet, however humble, and feel that
you regard him or her as a person of
importance.

Fruit Cocktail Cake

2 eggs, beaten
1½ c. sugar
Can fruit
2 c. flour
2 tsp. soda
Pinch of salt
⅔ c. nuts, chopped
½ c. brown sugar
½ c. Milnott
Stick oleo
¾ c. coconut
½ c. brown sugar
Stir together eggs, sugar, fruit, flour, soda, salt and pour into baking pan. Mix and pour over it the nuts, Milnott, oleo, coconut, and brown sugar. Bake at 350° F. for 25 minutes.
Frosting
1 c. sugar
½ c. Milnott
Stick oleo
¾ c. coconut
1 tsp. vanilla
Mix ingredients and pour over warm cake. Put back into the oven and brown slightly.
From the kitchen of Ethel A.

Mincemeat Cake

½ c. butter
1 c. white sugar
2 egg yolks, beaten
2 c. flour, sifted
½ tsp. soda
1½ tsp. baking powder
½ tsp. salt
1 c. raisins
1 lb. mincemeat
1 c. walnuts, chopped
1 tsp. vanilla
2 egg whites
Separate eggs.
Cream butter, sugar vanilla and two beaten egg yolks. Add flour, salt, soda, baking powder and mix well. Add raisins, mincemeat, and chopped walnuts. Fold in egg whites which have been beaten stiff but not dry. Bake in moderate oven (350° F.) for 1 hour.
From the kitchen of Imodean D.

"You are only young once, but you can be immature forever."
"I believe that our background and circumstances may have influenced who we are, but we are responsible for who we become."

Italian Cream Cake

2 c. sugar
½ c. shortening
1 stick oleo
5 eggs
2 c. flour, sifted
1 tsp. soda
1 c. buttermilk
1 - 8 oz. pkg. flaked coconut
Separate eggs. Beat egg whites. Cream together sugar, shortening and oleo. Add egg yolks and beat well. Add remaining ingredients. Fold egg whites into batter. Bake in 3 layers for 25 - 30 minutes at 350° F.
From the Kitchen of Imodean A.

Oatmeal Cake

1½ c. boiling water over 1 c. quick oats.
Cream:
1 c. brown sugar
1 c. white sugar
½ c. shortening
Add:
2 eggs
1 tsp. vanilla
1½ c. flour and pinch salt
1 tsp. soda
1 tsp. cinnamon
Mix the ingredients and cooked oatmeal. Bake at 325° F. about 40

minutes.
Icing:
6 tbsp. butter
⅓ c. cream
½ c. brown sugar.
Mix and bring to a boil.
Add:
1 c. coconut
½ c. nuts
Spread on warm cake and broil for one minute.
From the kitchen of Imodean A.

Peach Pound Cake

1 c. butter, softened
2 c. granulated sugar
6 eggs
1 tsp. almond extract
1 tsp. vanilla extract
3 c. all-purpose flour
¼ tsp. baking soda
¼ tsp. salt
½ c. sour cream
3 c. diced peaches, drained
Confectioners' sugar
Preheat oven to 350° F. Grease and flour a 10 inch fluted tube pan. Cream to together butter and granulated sugar in a large bowl. When light and fluffy, add eggs one at a time, beating after each addition. Stir in almond and vanilla extracts. In a separate bowl,

combine flour, baking soda and salt. Add flour mixture alternately with sour cream to creamed butter mixture. Fold in the peaches. Do not over-stir. Spoon into pan. Bake 55 - 65 minutes or until a tooth pick inserted in the center comes out clean. Cool 15 minutes before inverting onto plate. Dust with confectioners' sugar. Top with a light lemon glaze.

From the kitchen of Mildred A.

Mandarin Orange Cake and Icing

Pkg. Yellow Cake mix

4 eggs

1 c. Wesson Oil

16 oz. can mandarin oranges

Combine cake mix, oil and oranges with juice. Add eggs, one at a time, beating after each egg is added.

Check box for size of pan. Bake for 20-25 minutes. at 350° F. Let cool.

Icing:

20 oz. can crushed pineapples

Large pkg. instant vanilla pudding

mix

9 oz. Cool Whip

Small can coconuts

Mix pineapple and juice with coconut and dry vanilla pudding mix. Add Cool Whip. Spread on the cake.

From the kitchen of Phyllis T.

Todd Family Maple Chiffon Cake

2¼ cake flour (or 2 c. enriched all-purpose flour)

¾. c. granulated sugar

3 tsp. baking powder

1 tsp. salt

¾ c. brown sugar

½ c. salad oil

8 eggs (5 egg yolks and 8 egg whites)

¾ c. cold water

2 tsp. maple flavoring

½ tsp. cream of tartar

1 c. finely chopped California walnuts

Sift flour, granulated sugar baking powder, and salt in into a mixing bowl. Stir in brown sugar. Make a well in dry ingredients.   In this order, add salad oil, egg yolks, water, and flavoring. Beat until satin smooth. Combine egg whites and cream of tartar in a large mixing bowl. Beat until they form very stiff peaks. (Stiffer than for meringue or angle cake)   Pour egg yolk batter in thin stream over entire surface of egg whites, gently cutting and folding down, across bottom, up the side and over. Just until blended. Fold in nuts. Bake in ungreased 10 inch tube pan at 325° F. for 55 minutes. Invert pan on funnel or tall bottle; let cool thoroughly. To remove cake, loosen sides and around the tube with a knife; invert pan and if it does not have a "lift out" bottom, tap edge sharply on table. Frost with Golden Butter Frosting. This is a cake we all made often and entered in fairs.

From the kitchen of Melba R.

Salad Dressing Cake

2 c. flour
1½ tsp. baking powder
1½ tsp. soda
1 c. sugar
4 tbsp. cocoa
Mix together then add:
1 c. cold water
1 c. salad dressing (Miracle Whip)
2 tsp. vanilla

Mix together dry ingredients. Stir together water, salad dressing and vanilla. Stir the liquid into the dry ingredients in a baking pan and then bake for 35 minutes at 350° F.

Icing:

1 c. sugar
¼ c. cocoa
¼ c. milk
¼ c. butter

Boil one minute. Stir until partly cool. Add 2 teaspoon vanilla and spread on cake.

From the kitchen of Melba R.

June's Coffee Cake

Betty Crocker Yellow Cake mix
Small instant vanilla pudding
2 tbsp. flour
¾ c. Wesson oil
¾ c. water and 1 tsp. vanilla
4 unbeaten eggs
½ c. pecans or walnuts, chopped
2 tsp. cinnamon
1/3 c. brown sugar

Put above ingredients, except nuts, cinnamon and brown sugar, into large mixing bowl and beat for 8 minutes. This is important) While beating, grease and flour tube or bundt pan. Put chopped walnuts or pecans in the bottom of pan. In small bowl mix cinnamon and brown sugar. After batter is beaten for 8 minutes pour 1/3 over chopped nuts. Then sprinkle the brown sugar and cinnamon, mix carefully over the batter. Add 1/3 more batter and sprinkle with remaining brown sugar mix. Add remaining batter. Use spatula and run around middle of the cake to swirl brown sugar mix. Bake at 325° F. oven for 55 minutes. or until done. Cool slightly before removing from pan. Ice while warm.

Frosting:

1 c. powdered sugar
1 tsp. butter flavoring
1 tbsp. milk approximately

Mix together ingredients. Pour and let drizzle down sides and top of cake while still warm. Makes a thin frosting.

From the kitchen of June M. (Also Melba R. and Catherine G.)

Danish Coffee Cake

4 c. + flour for board
1 c. margarine
5 tbsp. sugar
1 tsp. salt
2 pkg. yeast
1 c. warm milk
2 eggs, beaten
3 cardamom seeds, crushed

Mix flour and margarine as for pie dough. Place yeast in warm milk and sugar. Add rest of ingredients and kneed together. Oil top and cover. Place in the refrigerator for 2 hours or overnight. Take out for refrigerator for 15-20 minutes before rolling out strips. Roll in 6 strips. Dot with butter and sprinkle with cinnamon, sugar, nuts around outer edges. Fold the edges over the sugar, cinnamon, nuts. Spread filling in the center. Fold over one side then the other in thirds. Place on greased pan and let rise 20 minutes. Beat one egg and spread over the tops. Sprinkle with cinnamon and sugar or apply an icing. Bake 15-20 minutes at 375° F. Frost and sprinkle with chopped nuts.

Filling:

1 lb. dates or dried apricots

1 c. sour cream

¼ c. light cream

1 c. sugar (optional: more or less)

Mix and boil and stir until smooth and thick - about 5 min.

Icing:

2 c. powdered sugar

¼ c. light cream

1 tsp. vanilla

Stir together and spread on the cake.

From the kitchen of Phyllis T.

Paula's Earthquake Cake

1 c. pecans, chopped

1 c. coconut flakes

Box German Chocolate Cake Mix

Small pkg. cream cheese

Stick soft margarine

Box powdered sugar

In the bottom of a 9 inch x 13 inch cake pan, mix cake mix according to the instruction on the box, and pour over pecans and coconut. Mix cream cheese, margarine and powdered sugar. Spread and swirl into German chocolate cake batter.

Bake at 350° F. for 50 minutes.

From the kitchen of Paula H.

Microwave Cherry Pudding Dessert Cake

Can (1 lb.6 oz.) prepared cherry pie filling
½ tsp. almond extract
½ c. butter or margarine
Pkg. (9 oz.) Layer Yellow Cake mix
1 c. chopped nuts

Mix together pie filling and almond extract in the bottom of a 9 in. round glass cake dish. In the bowl, cut butter into dry cake mix using a pastry blender or two knifes. Sprinkle over top on the pie filling along with nuts. Microwave on HI 12-15 minutes. Let stand 5 minutes. If desired, top with whipped cream or ice cream.

From the kitchen of Linda A.

Miracle Milnot Cheese Cake

3 oz. pkg. lemon jello
1 c. boiling water
3 tbsp. lemon juice
8 oz. cream cheese
1 c. sugar
1 tsp. vanilla
1 lb. graham crackers
½ c. melted oleo
Can chilled Milnot (or evaporated milk)

Dissolve lemon jello in the boiling water.

Add lemon juice. Cool. Cream together the cream cheese, sugar and vanilla and add to jello mixture. Whip chilled Milnot until peaks form. Fold gently into gelatin mixture. Mix melted oleo into 2/3 of the crushed crackers and pack 2/3s of them in the bottom and sides of a 9 x 13 x 1 inch pan. Add filling and sprinkle with remaining crushed crackers. Chill for 4-5 hours before serving.

From the kitchen of Sandra P.

Keep skid chains on your tongue. Always say less than you think. Cultivate a low, persuasive voice. How you say it often counts more that what you say.

Mc Call's Perfect Spice Cake

2¼ c. sifted cake flour

1 tsp. baking powder

¾ tsp. baking soda

1 tsp. salt

¾ tsp. cloves

¾ tsp. cinnamon

pinch of black pepper

¾ c. shortening, butter or margarine

¾ c. brown sugar, firmly packed

1 c. granulated sugar

1 tsp. vanilla extract, 3 eggs

1 c. buttermilk or sour milk

Assemble utensils and ingredients.

Start oven at 350° F. or moderate. Next heavily grease bottoms and sides of three 8-inch cake pans with shortening. (Do not use any salted fat) Then coat with flour. Dump out any surplus. This device help baked cakes drop from pan easily. Sift flour. Then spoon lightly into a standard measuring cup and cut off excess to make a level measurement. Do not shake flour into cup. Sift flour again this time with baking powder, soda, salt, cloves, cinnamon and pepper. Right here if your brown sugar is lumpy, sift or roll it. Now with your nice clean hands, work or cream the shortening, butter or margarine with a beating motion until it looks like whipped cream. At this point, begin to work in the brown sugar a little at a time, next the granulated sugar. Then add vanilla extract. Continue creaming until mixture is very fluffy and the grains of sugar almost disappear. This is a bit of a chore but it's the trick that makes a wonderful texture. When sugar is all in, add the eggs, unbeaten, one at a time, beating hard after each addition. From here on, work fast. Don't fool around. Now you begin to add the flour mixture. Sift about 1/8 cup into the batter and stir it in. Do not beat. Then add about ½ of the buttermilk or sour milk and stir it in. Repeat these operations ending with flour. Pour batter into greased pans, dividing it evenly. Bake 30 -35 min. or until cake edges leave sides of the pan. Remove from oven and let cool about 5 min. before turning out on a cake rake. This was a recipe that the Todd girls made many times for dessert and was entered in numerous fairs. This is the way the recipe directed in 1950's magazines. From the kitchen of Catherine G.

"I believe that our background and circumstances may have influenced who we are, but we are responsible for who we become."

Russian Bundt Cake

pkg. yellow cake mix (No
    pudding, not lemon)
6-oz. size chocolate instant pudding
1 c. oil
¾ c. water
½ c. sugar
4 eggs, beaten
¼ c. Kahlua
¼ c. vodka

Mix well with electric mixer for 2 minutes. Spray bundt pan with Baker's Joy, using it sparingly. Have oven heated to 350° F. Bake in the center of oven for 40 to 55 minutes. Test for doneness. Do not over

bake. Should still be moist.

Glaze:

¼ c. Kahlua

½ c. powdered sugar

A pastry brush is needed to apply the glaze while the cake is still hot. From the kitchen of Bobbye P.

Pillsbury Coconut Fluff Cake

Sift together:

1 tsp. salt

1¾ c. sugar

2½ c. Pillsbury flour

4½ tsp. baking powder

Add:

¾ c. vegetable shortening

11/8 c. milk

Beat for 2 minutes on medium speed until well blended.

Add:

2/3 c. egg whites, unbeaten

1 tsp. almond extract.

Beat for 2 minutes. Pour into two lightly greased 9 inch cake pans and bake at 350° F for 35 minute. From the kitchen of Irene T.

Mother's Coconut - Pineapple Cake

Yellow Cake Mix (without pudding)

Pkg. vanilla instant pudding

Can Eagle Brand Milk (not evaporated)

16½ can of crushed pineapple (drained)

1 c. cream of coconut

Mix vanilla pudding, cake, and milk together pour in a 9 x 12 oiled bottom pan. Bake according to directions on the cake mix box. While hot, punch holes in cake with fork. Then pour the cream of coconut over the cake. Spread crushed drained pineapple over the top of these. Let cool. Spread one container of whipped topping (small Cool Whip) over cake and sprinkle with coconut. Refrigerate. From the kitchen of Irene T.

Fig Cake

3 eggs

¾ c. vegetable oil

½ c. buttermilk

1 tsp. soda, dissolved in 2 tsp. water

2 c. all-purpose flour and 1 tsp. salt

1 tsp. ground cinnamon

1 tsp. ground nutmeg

1 tsp. ground allspice

1 tsp. vanilla extract

1 c. fig preserves with juice, chopped

1 c. chopped nuts

Powdered sugar

Beat eggs with electric mixer until thick and lemon colored; add sugar and oil, beating well. Combine buttermilk and soda. Sift next 5 ingredients together; add to egg mixture alternately with buttermilk mixture, mixing well after each addition. Stir in vanilla, figs, and nuts. Pour batter into a greased and floured 10 inch tube pan. Bake at 350° F. for 1 hour and 10 - 15 minutes. Cool 20 to 30 minutes. Remove from pan and sprinkle with powdered sugar. Serve.

From the kitchen of Lucille A.

to put them in hot water before you know how strong they are."

Mother's Seven Minute Icing

Seven Minute Icing
1 c sugar   2 egg whites
¼ C water   ¼ C Karo.
1 t Vanilla
Cook sugar, water + Karo for 7 minutes
over boiling beating constantly with a rotary
beater, Remove from stove add
Vanilla + beat until thick,

From the kitchen of Irene T.

June's Applesauce Cake

½ c. shortening

2 c. sugar

2 eggs

1 ½ c. applesauce

2 ½ c. flour

½ tsp. salt

½ tsp. cinnamon

½ tsp. cloves

½ tsp. all spice

1 c. raisins or dates (chopped)

½ c. chopped nuts

2 tsp. soda

½ c. boiling water

Cream shortening and add sugar gradually. Add eggs (well beaten) Stir in applesauce. Sift flour, spices and salt together. Take out 2 tablespoons of flour mixture and mix with dates and nuts. Dissolve soda in boiling water. Add sifted drying ingredients to creamed mixture. Then add soda water mixture to this. Stir in floured dates and nuts and mix well. Bake for 50 minutes at 350° F.

From the kitchen of June M.

Powder Sugar Icing

¼ c. shortening

½ c. brown sugar or white sugar

1 c. powdered sugar

2 tsp. chocolate (Cocoa)

Mix and cook for 2 minutes, then remove from the stove.

Add:

2 tsp. milk

Return to stove and bring to a boil for one minute. Let it cool and then spread it on the cake.

From the kitchen of Irene T.

Carmel Icing

1 c. sugar

½ c. cream

1 tsp. vanilla

Cook cream and sugar with pinch of soda until it forms a soft ball. Add vanilla.
Great for Angel Food Cakes.
From the kitchen of Melba R.

Golden Butter Frosting

½ c. butter or oleo
1 lb. (3½ c.) sifted confectioners' sugar
½ c. light cream
1 or 1½ tsp. maple flavoring or vanilla

Melt butter in saucepan, keep over low heat until golden brown, watching carefully so it doesn't scorch. Remove from heat and stir in confectioners' sugar. Blend in cream and flavoring. Place pan in ice water and beat until of spreading consistency (more cream may be added if needed). Makes enough to cover top and sides of 10 inch round chiffon or angel food cake.
From the kitchen of Melba R.

A true friend is someone who knows you're a good egg even if you're a little cracked.

Mother's Coconut Icing

1 tsp. oleo
1 c. sugar
1 c. water
1 tsp. vanilla
½ tsp. salt and pinch of tartar
Egg white
½ c. coconut

Make a syrup by boiling water, sugar, oleo and cream of tartar until it will form a soft ball in cold water. Beat egg white, add salt and pour syrup over egg white gradually. Add vanilla and beat until cool. Spread on the cake and sprinkle with coconut.
From the kitchen of Irene T.

Wilma's Carmel Icing

1½ c. brown sugar
6 tbsp. cream or milk
1½ c. powdered sugar
1 tbsp. oleo
1 tsp. vanilla

Bring to a boil the brown sugar and cream or milk. Add the powdered sugar, beat and add oleo and vanilla. Spread as soon as possible.
From the Kitchen of Wilma V.

German Chocolate Cake Icing

1 c. sugar
3 egg whites, beaten
Can angle flake coconut
1 tall can Pet milk
½ c. pecans
1 tsp. vanilla
1 stick oleo
Mix all ingredients together and cook on med heat until thick while stirring. Let cool before icing cake
From the kitchen of Irene T.

Sea Foam Frosting

2 eggs whites
1½ c. firmly packed dark brown sugar
1/3 c. water
1 tbsp. corn syrup
1 tsp. cream of tartar
1 tsp. vanilla extract
Combine first five ingredients in top of double boiler and beat for 1 minute. Place over boiling water and beat on high speed 7 minutes. Remove from double boiler and put in vanilla extract and beat another 2 minutes and it is ready. Ices two cakes.

Cream Cheese Frosting

Pkg. 8 oz. cream cheese, softened
½ c. butter, softened
1 lb. powdered sugar
1 tbsp. instant chocolate pudding
1 tsp. vanilla
Beat ingredients and spread on cool cake and refrigerate.
From the kitchen of Mildred A.

Easy Penache Icing

¼ c. Oleo
1 c. brown sugar
¼ c. milk
1¾ to 2 c. sifted confectioner's sugar
Melt oleo in sauce pan. Add brown sugar. Boil over low heat 2 minutes, stirring constantly. Stir in milk. Bring to a boil, stirring constantly. Cool to luke warm. Gradually add confectioner's sugar. Beat until thick enough to spread. If icing becomes too stiff, add a little warm water.
From the kitchen of Irene T.

Brown Sugar Icing

¼ c. oleo
2 tbsp. milk
½ c. brown sugar
1 c. powdered sugar
1 tsp. vanilla

Bring oleo and brown sugar to boil to dissolve sugar. Add milk and bring to a boil. Cool. Add powdered sugar and vanilla and beat. Let cool and spread on cake.
From the kitchen of Mopaul S.

Cheese Cake

(Bulk Recipe)

6 lb. cream cheese
Add:
2 oz. butter
1 lb. sugar
6 oz. cake flour
1 lemon juice
Add:
10 eggs
4 egg yolks
Add:
1 c. cream

Spread corn flake crumbs into your baking pan. Spread mixed ingredients over the crumbs.
From the Skirvin Tower Hotel, Oklahoma City, OK, 1960.

The people who make a difference in your life are not the ones with the most credentials, the most money, or the most awards. They are the ones that care.

Chocolate Cake and Icing

(Bulk Recipe)

Cake:

5 lb. cake flour
2 lb. cake shortening
1 lb. butter
6 lb. + 12 oz. sugar
1½ oz. salt
3 oz. soda
1 oz. baking powder
1 # cocoa
4 lb butter milk

Mix at 2d speed for 6 minutes, then at 1st speed for 4 minutes after adding the following.
3 lb. whole eggs and 3½ lb. butter milk

Icing:

Step 1, Boil together
1½ lb. milk
2 lb. sugar
Step 2, add:
10 lb. powdered sugar
½ tsp. vanilla
Pinch salt

Step 3, melt together:
1½ lb. shortening
1½ lb. butter
Step 4, add:
¾ c. Karo Syrup, dark
Step 5, melt and add:
1 to 1½ qt. Baker's chocolate
From the Skirvin Tower Hotel,
Oklahoma City, OK, 1960.

Orange Chiffon Cake and Icing

(Bulk Recipe)

Cake:

Blend by Sifting:
3 lb. 6 oz. cake flour
2 ¾ oz. baking powder
1¼ oz. salt
Add to Above:
3 lb. sugar
Mix and Add:
1 lb. + 1 oz. Wesson oil
1 lb. + 12 oz. egg yolks
1 lb. + 12 oz. water
Stir together and Add:
14 oz. orange juice
4 oz. grated orange rind
3 lb + 8 oz. egg whites
8 oz. cream of tartar
1 lb + 10 oz. sugar
1 lb + 12 oz. scalz

Icing:

10 lbs. powdered sugar
1 lb. powdered milk
5 lb. quick-blend shortening
1 lb. 8 oz. butter
½ oz. salt
Add:
2 oz. orange juice and 4 oz. orange rind (grated)
½ tsp. lemon powder
Add lightly:
1 lb. egg whites and 1 lb. 8 oz. water (variable) and Puri vanilla
From the Skirvin Tower Hotel, Oklahoma City, Oklahoma, 1960

Banana Cake

(Bulk Recipe)

Cream together:

4 lb. + 2 oz. sugar

2 lb. shortening

1 oz. soda

2 lb. eggs

Vanilla flavoring

1 ½ oz. salt

Add:

3 lb. + 4 oz. bananas

1 lb. + 12 oz. butter milk

3 lb. + 4 oz. cake flour

1 lb. + 3 oz. scalz

From the Skirvin Tower Hotel, Oklahoma City, OK, 1960.

White Cake

(Bulk Recipe)

5 lb. cake flour

3 lb. cake shortening

6 lb. + 4 oz. sugar

2 ½ oz. salt

2 oz. baking powder

8 oz. milk

½ oz. cream of tartar

2 ¾ lb. water

½ oz. cream of tartar

2 ¾ lb. water

Mix (at 2nd speed for 5 minutes) the above ingredients, then add and mix at 1st speed for 5 minutes.

Add:

3 lb. egg whites

8 oz. water

Bake at 350° F.

From the Skirvin Tower Hotel, Oklahoma City, OK, 1960.

New Kind of Drug: Hugging
Hugging Is Healthy

It helps the body's immune system. It keeps you healthier. It cures depression. It reduces stress. It induces sleep. It's invigorating. It's rejuvenating. It has no unpleasant side effects. Hugging is nothing less than a miracle drug. HUGGING IS NATURAL It is organic and naturally sweet. It has no pesticides, no preservatives and no artificial ingredients. It is 100 percent wholesome.
HUGGING IS PRACTICALLY PERFECT

God Has Hand in Our Lives

I asked God to take away my habit. God said, no. It is not for me to take away, but for you to give it up. I asked God to make my handicapped child whole. God said, no. His spirit is whole, his body is only temporary. I asked God to grant me patience. God said, no. Patience is a byproduct of tribulations; it isn't granted, it is learned. I asked God to give me happiness, God said, no. I give you blessings; Happiness is up to you. I asked God to spare me pain. God said, no. Suffering draws you apart from worldly cares and brings you closer to me. I asked God to make my spirit grow. God said, no. You must grow on your own, but I will prune you to make s you fruitful. I asked God for all things that I might enjoy life. God said, no. I will give you life, so that you may enjoy all things. I asked God to help me LOVE others, as much as He loves me. God said...Ahhhh, finally you have the idea.
Author Unknown

Chapter 12

Ice Cream

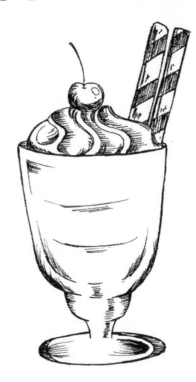

Index of Ice Cream Recipes

Zip Lock Shaker Ice Cream

In a pint zip lock bag, mix
½ c. milk
1 tbsp. sugar
½ tsp. vanilla
Seal. Place the pint bag into a gallon zip lock bag that has been half filled with five cups crushed ice and six tablespoons of salt. Seal. Shake 5-10 minutes, until desired consistency. Wipe off water on small bag before opening. Eat from the pint bag (with a spoon!). Makes a serving for one.
From the kitchen of Phyllis T.

Mr. Clapper's Peach Ice Cream

Small mixer bowl of peaches, chopped and sweeten to taste
3 eggs
2 c. sugar
Tall can of evaporated milk
pinch of salt
1 tsp. vanilla
Mix and pour into freezer canister. Add whole milk to fill line. Makes one gallon. Then follow the directions of your ice cream freezer.
From the kitchen of Mr. Clapper

Vanilla Ice Cream

6 eggs
1 qt. whipping cream
2 c. sugar
¾ c. white Karo syrup
13 oz. or 3 c. marsh mellow creme
4 tsp. vanilla
Salt to taste
Beat eggs until very thick and lemon colored. Add sugar gradually while beating. Add Karo and mix well. Stop mixer, add marsh mellow cream and beat slowly. Add whipping cream and vanilla and continue beating until well mixed. Add milk to make 1½ gallon. (May use less cream.)
From the kitchen of Phyllis T.

Home Made Ice Cream

6 eggs
3 c. milk
1 lg. can Pet Milk
2¼ c. sugar
2 tbsp. vanilla
dash of salt
1 pt. Half and Half

Beat the eggs. Scald the 3 cup milk and add to the eggs. Continue to beat while adding the Pet Milk. Add sugar, vanilla, salt, Half and Half and cream. Put in freezer bowl. Fill the bowl up with milk and freeze.
From the kitchen of Mildred A.

Little Green Things

3 oz. pkg. lime flavored gelatin
¾ c. sugar
Dash of salt
1 c. boiling water
1 c. cold water
6 oz. can (¾ c.) frozen limeade
    concentrated, thawed
1½ c. light cream
8 small cups
8 pop cycle sticks

In mixing bowl, combine gelatin, sugar and salt. Add boiling water; stir until gelatin and sugar are dissolved. Stir in cold water, limeade concentrate, and cream. Freeze until firm. With wooden spoons, break into chunks; with electric or rotary beater, beat until smooth. Quickly fill small paper cups and insert sticks. Freeze until firm. Makes about 8 servings. To serve, peel off paper cups. To make pink things, substitute pink lemonade and cherry flavored gelatin.
From the kitchen of Phyllis T.

Chocolate Ice Cream

1½ c. sugar
½ c. cocoa
Dash of salt
2½ tbsp. cake flour
2 c. milk
5 beaten eggs yolks
1 tsp. vanilla
½ c. sugar
5 beaten egg whites
Small can Hershey's chocolate syrup
Can Eagle brand milk
Large can Milnot
½ pint whipping cream, not whipped

Mix the dry ingredients. Add milk and egg yolks. Cook in top of double boiler, stirring constantly until thick. Cool. Add vanilla. Beat the egg whites until peaks form and gradually add sugar. Pour into one gallon freezer can. Mix in the chocolate mixture of Hershey's chocolate syrup, Eagle brand milk, Milnot and whipping cream.

From the kitchen of Phyllis T.

Rocky Road Fudge Bars

Bar: ½ c. margarine or butter
1 square (1 oz.) unsweetened chocolate or 1 envelope pre-melted, unsweetened baking chocolate flavor
1 c. sugar
1 c. Pillsbury's Best All Purpose or Unbleached Flour
1 tsp. baking powder
½ to 1 c. chopped nuts
1 tsp. vanilla
2 eggs

Filling:
8 oz. pkg. cream cheese, softened (Reserve 2 oz. for frosting)
½ cup sugar
2 tsp flour
¼ c. margarine or butter, softened
 ½ tsp vanilla
1 egg
¼ c. chopped nuts

6 oz. pkg. (1 c.) semi sweet chocolate chips if desired

Frosting:
2 c. miniature marsh mellows
¼ c. margarine or butter
1 square (1 oz.) unsweetened chocolate or 1 envelope pre-melted unsweetened baking chocolate flavor and 2 oz. reserved cream cheese
¼ c. milk
3 c. powdered sugar
1 tsp. vanilla

Heat oven to 350° F. Grease (not oil) and flour a 13 inch x 9 inch pan. In large saucepan over low heat, melt ½ cup margarine and 1 square chocolate (lightly spoon flour into measuring cup; level off.) Add remaining bar ingredients; mix well. Spread in prepared pan. In small bowl, combine 6 ounce cream cheese with next five Filling ingredients. Beat one minute at medium spread until smooth and fluffy; stir in nuts. Spread over chocolate mixture. Sprinkle with chocolate chips. Bake at 530° F for 25-30 minutes or until toothpick inserted in center comes out clean. Remove from oven; sprinkle with marsh mellows. Bake 2 minutes longer. In large saucepan, over low heat, melt ¼ cup margarine, one square chocolate, remaining two ounces cream cheese and milk. Stir in powdered sugar and vanilla until smooth. Immediately pour over marsh mellows and swirl together. Cool; cut into bars. Store in refrigerator. Makes 3-4 dozen bars. From the kitchen of Catherine G.

Hot Chocolate Sauce

2 sq. chocolate
16 marsh mellows
½ c. water
Stir together over low heat until marsh mellows and chocolate melt. Add these and stir.
½ c. sugar and ¼ tsp. salt
½ tsp. vanilla
Let cool slightly and serve over ice cream.

From the kitchen of Linda A.

Goodie Freezer Bars

¾ c. instant dry milk
1½ c. water
1½ c. peanut butter (smooth or chunky)
Pkg. chocolate instant pudding
1 lb. box graham crackers
Mix instant milk and water   Add peanut butter and beat together until well mixed.   Add instant pudding and stir until smooth. Spread generously on a graham cracker and top with another graham cracker, sandwich style. Repeat until all the filling is used. Freeze in a tight container. These may be eaten immediately when removed from the freeze.
From the kitchen of Linda A.

Chapter 13
Candy Recipes

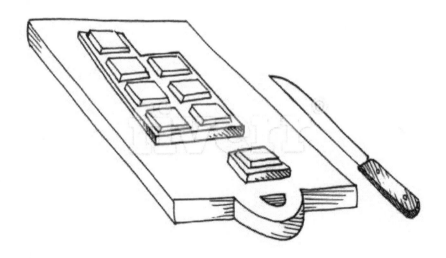

Lewis A. and Linda J. Armstrong

Index of Candy Recipes

3 Minute Microwave Fudge

½ c. margarine (1 stick)
½ to 1 c. of pecans or walnuts, chopped
½ c. cocoa
¼ c. evaporated milk
1 tsp. vanilla
1 - 1 lb. box of powdered sugar
Melt margarine in glass bowl in the microwave. Add cocoa, milk, and powdered sugar. Stir. Cook for 2 minutes in microwave on full power. Stir and cook for 1 more minutes. Stir in nuts and vanilla. Pour into buttered 9-inch x 9-inch pan, cool, and cut.
From the kitchen of Linda A.

Chocolate Fudge

2½ c. white sugar
½ c. dark Karo syrup
3 tbsp. cocoa
1¼ c. whipping cream
½ c. nuts, chopped
1 tbsp. vanilla
Stir together sugar, syrup cocoa, and cream and cook until forms semi firm hard ball in cool water, then remove from the fire and beat until very thick. Add nuts and vanilla. Pour in buttered pan and cut in squares.
From the kitchen Pearl Y., Laing Community and Linda A.

Chocolate Fudge

2 c. sugar
1 c. of canned milk
2 squares chocolate
2 tbsp. Karo
2 tbsp. of oleo
1 c. pecans, chopped
Combine milk, sugar, chocolate, and Karo. Cook on stove top to 232° F. Remove from burner and add butter and pecans. Beat until it gets firm enough to pour into a buttered 9-inch x 13-inch pan. Cut when cool.
From the kitchen of Irene T.

Velveeta Cheese Fudge

2 sticks oleo
½ lb. Velveeta cheese
½ c. cocoa
1 c. nut
1 tsp. vanilla
2 lb. bag powdered sugar
Melt the oleo. Add cheese and stir over low heat until melted. Add cocoa, nuts, vanilla, and powdered sugar. Mix till smooth. Spread in 9-inch x 13-inch pan. Refrigerate.
From the kitchen of Veletta A.

Marshmellow Cream Fudge

5 c. sugar

Can of evaporated milk

3 small pkg. of chocolate chips (18 oz.)

13 or 8 oz. jar marsh mellow cream

1 lb. of pecans (2 c.)

1 - 2 tsp. vanilla

1/8 lb. of butter or oleo (2 oz.) (1/2 Stick or in saucepan

Mix sugar and milk together. Place on burner, stirring all the time at a med-low heat. When it starts boiling good, start timing and boil slowly 8 minutes. Remove from fire. Add chocolate chips, cream, butter and vanilla. Beat this until it is stiff enough to pour in a buttered pan. Just before pouring out, add pecans. Makes 5 pounds of more.

From the kitchen of Aunt Thel H. and Irene T.

Never put both feet in your mouth at the same time, because then you won't have a leg to stand on.

Grudge Fudge

12 oz. pkg. chocolate chips

1 c. butter (Two Sticks)

2 eggs

1 lb. pkg. powdered sugar

½ tsp. vanilla

1 c. chopped nuts of choice

Melt chocolate chips and butter over hot not boiling water. In mixing bowl, beat eggs until lemon in color and lightly thick. Add powdered sugar, adding a small amount at a time, beating constantly till smooth. Add chocolate mix. Add vanilla and nuts and mix well. Pour into 8-inch x 8-inch pan and cover with saran wrap. Refrigerate until set

.

"I started out with nothing and I still have most of it."

Never take life seriously. Nobody gets out alive anyway.

Microwave Million Dollar Fudge

4½ c. sugar
7 oz. jar marsh mellow crème
13 oz. can of Pet Evaporated Milk
1 stick margarine and 1 tsp. vanilla
3 giant Hershey Bars (24 oz. total)
1 lb. coarsely chopped nuts (3 c.)
12 oz. pkg. Nestle Chocolate
     Morsels

In a microwave, melt chocolate morsels and bars for about 2½ minutes each. Remove lid and melt marshmallow cream in the jar for 25 seconds. Butter (or lightly spray with Pam) one 8 inch square glass pan and a 2 or 3 quart oblong, utility dish. Use more pans--depending on thickness desired. Combine sugar, milk, and margarine in a deep (3 quart) bowl and stir to blend. Microwave on HI for 11 to 13 minutes. Stir to keep from boiling over till a small amount dropped in a cup of cold water forms a soft ball or check with candy thermometer for soft ball stage. Remove from oven and add all remaining ingredients. Pour into prepared pans. Let stand for at least 24 hours. Great for Christmas - make early and freeze in metal tins.
From the kitchen of Mrs. Aschbacher

7 Pound Christmas Fudge

3 large bars (8 oz. each) milk
     chocolate, broken in small pieces
2 pkg. (11.5 oz.) Milk chocolate bits
Large jar (13 oz.) Marshmallow
     cream
4 c. sugar
Tall can (13 oz.) evaporated milk
½ lb. butter
2 tsp. vanilla
1 c. black walnuts or pecans,
     chopped

In a large mixing bowl of heavy duty electric mixer, combine broken chocolate bars, chocolate bits and marshmallow crème; set aside. In large, heavy saucepan, combine sugar, evaporative milk and butter. Cook and stir over medium heat until mixture boils: boil 5 minutes. Pour hot mixture over chocolate mixture. Beat until ingredients are thoroughly blended, beat in vanilla. Remove beaters and stir in chopped nuts. Quickly pour mixture into buttered 9-inch x 13-inch x 2-inch pan. Cool. Cover tightly and refrigerate until firm enough to cut into small squares. Flavors will be best after a week of storage.
From the kitchen of Mildred A.

Chocolate Marshmellow Fudge

4½ c. sugar and ½ c. butter or oleo
2½ pkgs. Chocolate chips
2 lg. Hershey's Bars
1 lg. can Pet Milk
8 oz. marshmallow whip
Boil sugar, milk and butter for eight minutes. Add rest of ingredients after pan in removed from the stove. Beat in chocolate and marshmallow. Candy will be soft. Pour into a greased jelly roll pan. Cool. Makes five pounds.
From the kitchen of Mildred A.

Kathy's Candy

7 oz. pkg. coconut
½ can sweetened condensed milk
Pkg. confectioner's sugar (1 lb.)
Stick oleo and 2 c. pecans
Mix ingredients and form into about sixty balls and freeze or refrigerate.
½ block paraffin
½ small pkg. chocolate chips
Melt paraffin and chips. Dip balls in melted chocolate and paraffin.
Makes about 60 balls
From the kitchen of Melba R.

Mother's Divinity

(L A's Favorite)

2 c. white sugar
¾ c. white Karo syrup
¼ c. boiling hot water
2 egg whites, beaten
½ c. nuts
Boil sugar and syrup until it spins a thread. Add stiffly beaten egg whites and nuts. Stir until it begins to harden. Pour into buttered tin and let set until it has hardened.
From the kitchen of Irene T.

Divinity

2 2/3 c. sugar and ½ c. of water*
2/3 c. light corn syrup
2 egg whites
1 tsp. vanilla
2/3 c. of broken nuts
   Stir sugar corn syrup and water over low heat until sugar is dissolved. Cook without stirring to 260° F. on candy thermometer (or until small amount of mixture dropped into very cold water forms a hard ball.) In mixer bowl, beat egg whites until stiff peaks form. Continue beating while pouring hot syrup in a thin stream into egg whites. Add vanilla; beat until

mixture holds its shape and becomes slightly dull. (Mixture may become too stiff for mixer.) Fold in nuts. Drop mixture from tip of buttered spoon onto waxed paper. About 4 dozen candies. *Use 1 tablespoon less water on a humid day.

From the kitchen of Karen R.

Microwave Peanut Brittle

1 c. sugar and 1 c. light corn syrup
1 tbsp. butter or margarine
1/8 tsp. salt
1 tsp. vanilla
1 to 1½ c. roasted, salted peanuts
1 tsp. baking soda

Combine sugar, syrup, and salt in 2-quart casserole or mixing bowl. Microwave 5 min. on HI. Stir in peanuts. Microwave 3 to 5 minutes HI, stirring after 3 minutes, till syrup and peanuts are lightly browned. Stir in butter, vanilla, and baking soda until light and foamy. Spread to ¼ inch thickness on large well-buttered cookie sheet. For very thin peanut brittle---cool mixture on cookie sheet for 3 to 5 minutes and then lift from sheet and pull or stretch mixture to desired thinness.

From the kitchen of Linda A.

Peanut Brittle

1½ c. sugar
1 c. white corn syrup
½ c. water
1/8 tsp. salt
1 pint raw peanuts
½ tsp. soda

Cook the sugar, syrup and water until it makes a hard ball when put in water. Add salt. Add peanuts and cook slowly until peanuts are roasted, almost ten minutes, but don't let syrup darken. Add soda. Mix quickly. Pour on a hard surface that has been greased in a little spot about the size of a saucer and not too thick. When cool enough, pull on the edges to stretch it out.

From the kitchen Aunt Thel H.

Spiced Walnuts

1 c. sugar
¼ tsp. salt
1 tsp. cinnamon
1¼ tsp. vanilla
7 tbsp. water
2 c. walnuts

Mix all but walnuts. Cook to soft ball stage without stirring. Remove from heat and dump in walnuts. Stir gently until syrup sugars. Pour onto greased pan and separate.

Cream Nut Loaf

3 c. white sugar
½ c. dark Karo
1½ c. sweet cream (whipping cream)
Cook together until forms semi hard ball. (Soft on the inside, firm on the outside.)
Remove from the stove and beat until creamy.

Add:

1 tbsp. vanilla
1½ c. nuts (peanuts, pecans, or walnuts)
Continue beating until very thick.
Pour in buttered pan and cut in squares when cool.
From the kitchen of Pearl Y.

Mother's Date Loaf Candy

3 c. sugar
1 c. rich milk
2 c. chopped dates
1 ½ c. nuts (chopped)
Place sugar and milk in a sauce pan. Stir over a low flame/heat until sugar is dissolved; increase the heat and boil to 238° F. (The soft ball stage) Add the dates and cook to 242° F. (Two or three minutes additional boiling.) Remove from the stove: cool, beat until candy begins to thicken. Add nuts and continue beating until the mixture is firm enough to form into a roll about an inch in diameter. Wrap in a wet cloth and let stand until thoroughly cold. Refrigerate. Remove cloth and cut into slices. The candy can be rolled into chopped nuts or shredded coconut before slicing. Makes 2 pounds. (Our mother made this in a big iron skillet.)
From the kitchen of Allene S.

Microwave Caramel Corn

½ c. butter (1 stick)
1 c. brown sugar
¼ c. light corn syrup
Dash salt
1 tsp. baking soda
12 c. popped corn (2 bags)
Pop corn in microwave, pour in brown paper bag. In large bowl, combine first four ingredients. Microwave 2 minutes. Stir. Microwave for an additional 3 minutes. Stir in soda and vanilla. Pour over popcorn in brown bag and stir well.
From the kitchen of Linda Y.

Candy Bars

1 c. brown sugar
1 c. butter of soft spread for
cooking
1 c. chopped pecans
3 c. crushed graham crackers
Line a cookie sheet with parchment
or with aluminum foil. Then in it,
pour as many of the crushed
graham crackers as possible,
spreading them across the lined
cookie sheet.   Stir together the
brown sugar and butter or soft
spread and bring to a boil in a sauce
pan. Add in the pecans. Bake in
an oven at 350° F. for ten minutes.
Cool, cut up, and place in sealed bag
to remain crisp.
From the kitchen Allene S.

Pearl's Coconut Candy

Cocoanut Candy   Pearl young's

1½ boxes Powdered sugar
I can Eagle brand milk   1t Vanilla
2 cans bakers cocoanut   2 c choped nuts
mix together and drop on waxed paper
and let stand in ref. over night. Melt
I large pkg. of chocolate chips (semi-
sweet) with ¼ lb parfin + dip the
1st part + place on waxed paper.

From the kitchen of Pearl Y.

Chapter 14

Appendix of Useful Information

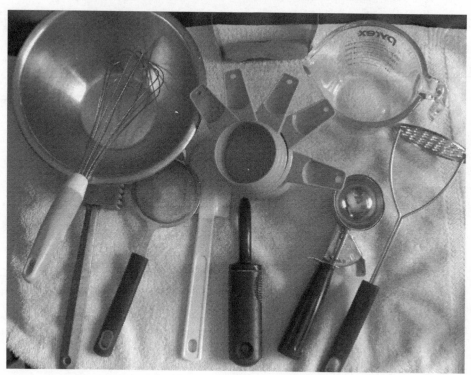

Appendix Index of Contents

SEASONINGS: TRY DIFFERENT VEGETABLE SEASONINGS

When trying a new herb, spice, or seasoning, use c to ¼ teaspoon of the ingredient per 1 c. of vegetable, until you decide if you like the flavor. Use cheeses, sour cream, horseradish, mustard, etc., in sauces to accompany vegetables. Cracker crumbs, nuts, olives, and other foods add interesting textures and flavors to vegetables. Here's a list of "flavor ideas'" to use as a seasoning guide. Try just one suggestion at a time to see if you like it – then use your imagination and taste buds as your guide.

SEASONING SUGGESTIONS:

ASPARAGUS--cheese, hard-cooked eggs, lemon juice

BEETS--honey, orange juice, celery seeds, allspice

BROCCOLI--cheese, nutmeg, mustard, almonds

BRUSSEL SPROUTS--sautéed cracker crumbs, cheese, nuts, lemon juice

BUTTER BEANS--onions, catsup, brown sugar

CARROTS--honey, mint, basil, brown sugar, pecans

CAULIFLOWER--pimento, cheese, mustard

CORN--sour cream, curry, chives, tomatoes, onions

GREEN BEANS--bacon, sautéed cracker crumbs, dill weed, nutmeg, almonds

LIMA BEANS--thyme, cheese, basil, pimiento

MIXED VEGETABLES--sour cream, parsley, chives, poppy seeds

PEAS--bacon, basil, onions, pimento, sour cream, horseradish

PEAS & CARROTS--basil, cheese, dill weed, onions

PORK & BEANS--catsup, barbeque spice, curry, maple syrup

POTATOES--parsley, poppy seeds, cheese, dill, chives

PUMPKIN--cinnamon, nutmeg, orange juice, rum, pecans

RED BEANS--celery seeds, sour cream, chives, savory, pimento

SAUERKAUT--caraway seeds, applesauce, mustard

SPINACH--sour cream, vinegar, bacon, hard-cooked eggs, nutmeg

SQUASH (WINTER)--dates, orange juice, raisins, cinnamon, allspice

SUCCOTASH--curry, savory, chicken bouillon, poultry seasoning

TOMATOES--oregano, basil, dill, sour cream, celery, celery seeds, chives

SIMPLIFIED MEASURES

dash or pinch = less than 1/8 teaspoon

2 pints (4 cups) = 1 quart

3 teaspoons = 1 tablespoon

4 quarts (liquid) = 1 gallon

16 tablespoons = 1 cup

8 quarts (solid) = 1 peck

1 cup = ½ pint

4 pecks = 1 bushel

2 cups = 1 pint

16 ounces = 1 pound

If you want to measure part-cups by tablespoon, remember:

4 tablespoons = ¼ cup

10 2/3 tablespoons = 2/3 cup

5 1/3 tablespoons = 1/3 cup

12 tablespoons = ¾ cup

8 tablespoons = ½ cup

14 tablespoons = 7/8 cup

Author Unknown

Oven Temperatures

Slow. . . . . .250 to 300 degrees

Slow moderate. . . . . .325 degrees

Moderate. . . . .350 degrees

Quick moderate. . . . . .375 degrees

Moderately hot. . . . . .400 degrees

Hot. . . . . .425 to 450 degrees

Very hot. . . . . .475 to 500 degrees

Estimate for Measuring

1 pound shell walnuts makes 4 cups of chopped nuts

22 vanilla wafers makes 1 cup finely crushed wafers

14 square graham crackers makes 1 cup fine crumbs

1 cup macaroni makes 2 cups cooked

16 ounce cheddar cheese makes 4 cups shredded cheese

1 cup long grain rice makes 3 cups cooked rice

1 cup package precooked rice makes 2 cups cooked rice

1 cup whipping cream makes 2 cups whipped cream

All Purpose Cleaner

(Use instead of Shout or Spray and Wash)

1 c. liquid dishwasher soap

1 c. ammonia

1 - 16 oz. bottle of alcohol

Mix all in 1 gallon jug and fill the rest with water. Put in a trigger spray bottle.

From the kitchen of Pat J.

HOUSEHOLD TIPS

Household Tip 1:   A great copper cleaner is a pinch of salt and the juice from half a lemon.

Household Tip 2:   Commercial, re-freezable, frozen "blue ice" is excellent for restoring carpet surface where table or other furniture has pressed down the carpet and pad. Lay a package of frozen blue ice on the spot and allow it time to thaw. Pick it up and you'll be surprised at the result. Re-freeze and use on other locations.

Household Tip 3:   A great carpet spot remover is 1 part white vinegar and 8 parts water. Use a soft <u>white</u> cloth dampened in the mixture, and blot away the spot. Then use a clean white cloth to blot the spot dry.

*Test the mixture on an out of the way area of the carpet to see if any color damage might possibly occur.

Household Tip 4:   TSP (Tri-sodium phosphate) is an excellent cleaning solution for cleaning hard to remove marks and stains on painted walls and wood work. Follow with clean water wipe down. TSP may be purchased at a hardware store. Use plastic gloves.

Household Tip 5:   Borax crystals are an excellent agent for eliminating fleas from pets as well as killing several other small household pests.

Sprinkle crystals over your carpet and in the sides and behind the cushions of your sofa and chairs.   Within a few days they will be gone.   It is harmless to your pets while also killing any fleas on your pets.

Household Tip 6:   Use this to polish you furniture. 1 part lemon juice and 2 parts vegetable oil. Mix it up and your house will look and smell lemony fresh.

Household Tip 7:   For a super drain cleaner, try antacid tablets, vinegar and hot water. Drop 2-3 antacid tablets in the drain, followed by a cup of white vinegar. After about five minutes, run the hot water for 3-4 minutes. No plumber, no big repair bill.

Household Tip 8:   For a dry carpet cleaner, create a powder mixture of ½ cup of cornstarch, 2 cups of baking soda, 1 tablespoon. Ground cloves and 4-5 crumbled bay leaves. Dust the carpet thoroughly then wait an hour before vacuuming. Author unknown.

20 USEFUL KITCHEN TIPS

Here are a few tried-and-true easy ideas for saving time and your energy(and maybe even your sanity!) in the kitchen!

1. When a bottle of corn syrup or pancake syrup is almost empty and that last bit is taking forever to come out-- just warm it in the microwave for a few seconds. It will be thinner and it will run right out!

2. When a recipe says to cover with aluminum foil while baking, just turn a cookie sheet upside down over the dish. Saves time and foil!

3. If your bananas begin to turn brown before you can use them, put them in the fridge! The skins will turn really brown, but the inside will stay fresh for several more days.

4. To make uniform sized muffins in a hurry, use an ice cream scoop to fill the cups. It is also lots neater!

5. To get that onion smell out of your hands after you've been peeling and chopping onions, sprinkle table salt on your hands and rub them together. Wash with soap and water and the smell will be gone!

6. Did you know that any brand of bottled Italian Salad Dressing makes a good marinade for meat?

7. When browning ground beef, try using a pastry blender to break the meat into smaller pieces. It works much better than a fork.

8. Canned chicken broth is a very tasty addition to any canned vegetable, instead of water. You might want to use the fat-free version.

9. Hate to spend the time it takes to clean that crock pot with the baked-on food? Line your slow-cooker with foil before adding recipe ingredients and clean up is a snap!

10. To make all your pancakes the same size, use your gravy ladle to pour the batter!

11. Your potato masher will mash bananas for banana bread or avocados

for guacamole in a hurry!

12. Buy several oranges and lemons when they are on sale. Put them in the freezer in zip-top bags. When a recipe calls for juice, just defrost in the microwave. When a recipe calls for grated peel, it's easy to grate while frozen.

13. Add a dash of vinegar to the water when boiling cabbage. You won't taste it, but it will cut down on the strong aroma

14. For easier, faster grating, store fresh ginger in the fridge.

15. Use your bottle brush or a clean old toothbrush to clean the grater after grating onions or cheese. Much faster and no more scraped hands!

16. To easily remove marshmallow creme from the jar, dip your spoon or knife in hot water first.

17. For easy-to-peel baked sweet potatoes, rub the skin with vegetable oil before baking. The skins will come right off.

18. Peel your vegetables over a half sheet of newspaper. When you're finished, just fold up and throw it all away!

19. To keep your graham cracker pie crust from getting soggy, be sure to use only butter or regular margarine. Don't use the new low-fat spreads. You can also bake it to keep it crisp. Just let it cool before adding filling.

20. When broiling meat, put ½ cup of water in the drip pan. There will be no smoke and cleanup is a snap!

Author unknown

ABOUT THE AUTHORS

Linda and Lewis were married June 1, 1963, in the building of the church of Christ in Tipton, Oklahoma. They celebrated their 50th Wedding Anniversary in 2013 in Fairbanks, Alaska. They have a son, Michael, and a daughter, Melinda. Linda has a degree in Vocational Home Economics from Oklahoma State University. Lewis graduated from Oklahoma State University and University of Kansas with degrees in Geography. He also has Masters in Library Science from Emporia State University and in Strategic and Political Studies from the Navy War College. He retired from the U.S. Army as a Colonel on December 31, 1993 at Fort Sam Houston, Texas. He has worked at three university libraries, University of Kansas, Abilene Christian University and Emporia State University, retiring from the latter in June 2003. In 2005 they moved to Georgia and have lived there since.

Other Books on Amazon

Books Written and Published

Stories by an Oklahoma Boy

Compiled and edited books on Amazon:

The Writings of Leonard E. Armstrong
Oh No, Another Email Story about Seniors
Oh No, Another Email Story about Relationships
Oh No, Another Email Story about Marriage and Family
Oh No, Another Email Story about Religion, Vol. 1
Oh No, Another Email Story about Religion, Vol. II
Oh No, Another Email Story about Individual Relationships
Oh No, Another Email Story about Holidays
Oh No, Another Email Story about Miscellaneous Stuff

Other Books in the works:

An autobiography titled: *An Oklahoma Boy on the Bumpy Road of Life*
An Armstrong Ancestry, first done by Elmo Armstrong
Love Letters During the Fog of the Vietnam War
A children's book: *The Boy that Dreamed*

Todd Family and Friends' Cookbook